January 11, 1978

2 sup.

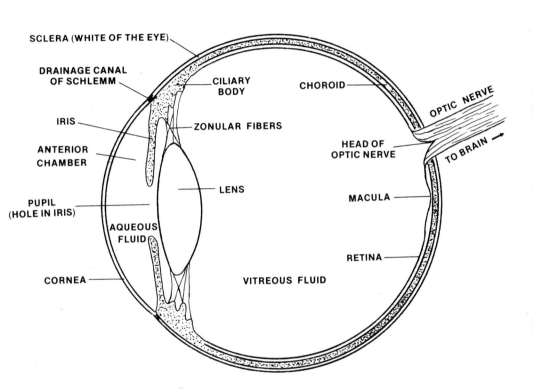

A CROSS SECTION OF THE EYE

10·25·77

The
Eye
Book

The Eye Book

Ben Esterman, M.D.

A Specialist's Guide to
Your Eyes and Their Care

Great Ocean Publishers
Arlington, Virginia

For information write

Great Ocean Publishers
738 South 22nd St.
Arlington, Virginia 22202

Distributed to the book trade by
Whirlwind Book Co.
80 Fifth Ave
New York City, New York 10011

Cover design by Pat Taylor

First Printing

Library of Congress Cataloging in Publication Data

Esterman, Ben.
  The eye book.

  Includes index.
  1. Eye—Care and hygiene.   2. Eye—Diseases
and defects.   I. Title.
RE51.E87   617.7   77-11660

ISBN 0-915556-04-9 (hardcover)
      0-915556-03-0 (paperback)

Manufactured in the United States of America

Contents

S 1983781

Acknowledgments

It is an accepted fact that one learns best by teaching. I am grateful to my students and to my patients, whose provocative questions over the years have laid the foundation for this book.

I am indebted to my secretaries, Mrs. Mary L. Spina for typing the several revisions of the manuscript and proofreading, and Mrs. Pearl Porter for her assistance; to Mrs. Julia Cahn for the final proofreading; and to my publisher for performing the innumerable tasks required in the production of an effective volume.

My wife, Cinabelle Morris Esterman, to whom this book is gratefully dedicated, devoted unlimited time and patience to editing, indexing, and above all to helping to translate the inevitably technical and scientific writing into language more comprehensible to the non-medical reader.

Preface

In the battle to cure or prevent disease, the cooperation of the informed and intelligent patient often makes the difference between success and failure. In dealing with eyes, this can mean sight or blindness.

Fortunately for patient and doctor alike, today's public wants to be informed. No longer is the modern patient content with receiving a prescription and directions. He isn't trying to be a doctor; he is seeking to learn something about his condition, about what's wrong and what can be done to correct it. By becoming informed, he helps himself and his doctor.

This book is **not** a "do-it-yourself" manual. It is not a substitute for competent professional service. It does not make suggestions for treatment of individual cases. It does dispel myth and misinformation and tries to supply facts which will alert the intelligent reader to the need for early help to avert illness or even blindness.

Much of the book is a summary in print of the simple, non-technical answers I have been giving to thousands of intelligent patients for over thirty years. Whatever success I have had in helping them I owe in part to their informed cooperation. It is at the suggestion of many of them, as well as of former students, that I write this for a larger audience.

No attempt has been made to cover the entire subject. That would take a hundred volumes of this size. To keep the book small I have dealt only with topics which interest the majority of patients and beg forgiveness of those whose favorite diseases I have omitted.

The need to simplify, even to oversimplify, is obvious. To make up for it, I have relegated to the final chapters the explanations of technical matters and terms, as well as descriptions and diagrams of the structure (anatomy) of the eye and how it works (physiology). Those wishing fuller understanding would do well to familiarize themselves with Chapter 16 on how the eye works and then refer to it again whenever suggested in the text. Frequent reference to the schematic diagram inside the front cover will also help the reader become oriented and familiar with the eye.

There is another reason for this book. I have found that young people are often fascinated by the few explanations they get in the course of an eye examination — sufficiently to arouse their curiosity and their desire to look further into the wonders of the eye. Over the years, a number of younger eye specialists have introduced themselves to me at professional meetings in distant places to say that their first interest in ophthalmology was awakened during visits to my office as patients while they were still in grade school.

It is my hope that young people reading this book, perhaps as a supplement to studies in science, will be "turned on" to learn more about their miraculous organ of sight. For a few it may even lead to a career.

Lawrence, N.Y.
May 4, 1977

1
"Doctor, Do I Need Glasses?"

Whether or not to wear glasses is the question which has caused more confusion than any other phase of eye care. Yet, the facts are quite simple and sensible. One does not need to be an eye specialist to understand them. Here are the questions patients ask most frequently:

Should I wear glasses?
If I should, must I wear them constantly?
Do I hurt my eyes by not wearing glasses?
    You will understand better if I answer the last question first. The answer is "No." Except for children with a tendency to a "lazy" eye, no one ever **harms** his eyes by **not** wearing his glasses. Blurring? Possibly. Discomfort? Perhaps. Harm? Definitely, no. Even if your vision is very blurred without glasses, or if removing them makes you uncomfortable, you still do no **harm** to your eyes by not wearing them.
    Just as not wearing glasses does no harm, wearing them does not cure anything or prevent anything, except for the conditions in children mentioned above. When you wear glasses you may see better or you may feel more comfortable; you do not change your eyes in any way. When you remove the glasses, your eyes remain exactly as they were before — no better, no worse. I often use the analogy of the woman with the high heeled shoes: when she wears them, all that happens is that she is a bit taller. The high heels cause no

permanent change in her height; neither do glasses change your eyes.

Now for the first two questions:

Should I wear glasses?
If I should, must I wear them constantly?

For a surprising number of people the answer to both questions is "No." For yourself, as an individual, it obviously depends on the condition of your eyes and on the way you use them. A specific answer, in your own case, can be given only after a careful examination by a competent professional.

In general, however, it is a fact that an incredible number of people wear glasses needlessly. Some wear them constantly although they really require them only for special occasions. Others wear them although they do not need to at all.

Glasses are worn for any of four reasons:
1. To see better
2. To see more comfortably
3. To protect the eyes in hazardous occupations
4. To help correct a crossed eye or "lazy" eye in childhood.

The fourth reason is discussed fully in Chapter 5; the third in Chapter 8. Only (1) and (2) need concern us here.

1. To see better:

Perfect (20/20) vision is very desirable — without glasses if you are lucky, with glasses if you cannot see adequately without them. But there is no rule that every human being must see 20/20 **all of the time.** People in certain special occupations obviously need accurate vision — the pilot, proofreader, surgeon, jeweler, seamstress, and the like — but only when they are at work. The same is true, though to a lesser degree, in less demanding pursuits — such as driving, reading, theater, school, television, — where vision ought to be adequate but not necessarily perfect. In any of these situations, whether you should wear glasses will depend entirely on how poor your vision is without them and how much sharpness your given task requires. In other words, the decision to wear or not to wear them can easily be made by you. The only exceptions are the requirements of the law for obvious reasons of public safety — that the pilot see 20/20 and the motor vehicle operator at least 20/40.

2. To see more comfortably

Some people see quite sharply without their glasses but are uncomfortable when they do not wear them. Discomfort may be felt as pain in the eyes, the brows, or the head. They may scowl, squint or frown. The eyes or lids may be red or teary, tired or heavy or sensitive to light. (Warning: all these could also be caused by certain eye diseases.)

Such discomfort may vary in different persons from slight to severe and may be constant or present only while using the eyes.

Here again, whether or not to wear glasses for discomfort depends on you — how much discomfort without them and how much relief with them.

Don't I strain my eyes by not wearing glasses?

Perhaps. At this point it is important to understand the meaning of "strain." "Strain" or "eyestrain" is not by itself a disease and is not physical damage. It is merely a symptom, something of which you may be aware within yourself. It usually appears as eye fatigue, burning, heaviness, tearing, sensitivity to light, a sandy sensation, blurring, even pain in the eyes or headache. Any one or combination of the above can be caused by a need for glasses. In such cases the proper glasses may give relief, which may justify their use whenever there is discomfort.

Are there other reasons for eyestrain beside the need for glasses?

Yes, indeed. It is important to keep in mind that your eyes are only part of the rest of you, and that they may be the first to show signs of trouble elsewhere. Whatever affects the rest of you can affect your eyes. Thus eye fatigue or strain, in the absence of a need for glasses, is often the result of general body fatigue, lack of sleep, general debility, emotional stress, frustration, even too sedentary an existence or lack of exercise. And a number of physical, ocular or general diseases may have eyestrain as one symptom. (See also Chapter 11 on your eyes and your health.) This is where the medical eye specialist comes in. It is he who not only determines whether there is a need for glasses but also, after a careful medical examination of the eyes, whether or not there is a disease or other condition which requires treatment, and how to treat it.

Do you really mean that lack of exercise can be a cause of eyestrain?

Definitely. I have helped many patients with eyestrain by correcting this factor alone, when there is no other cause. Let me give you a typical example from my files: A 32 year old man visited me a year ago complaining of eye strain. Six months earlier someone in a department store had sold him "rest glasses" which had not helped. Thorough examination of his eyes revealed no disease and no need for glasses.

I questioned him about his work and his habits. He was a full-time accountant, spent his evenings reading or watching television. He was completely sedentary, drove to work, did not even have a dog to walk and, though medically normal, was about thirty pounds overweight.

I explained how the eyes are part of the body, and that they fatigue more easily when the general body tone is poor. And I pointed out that he was spending his evenings doing more of what he did all day long — using his eyes at close range. While he was doing no physical damage he was creating an inordinate amount of fatigue.

I suggested he put away his glasses until he was forty, and make no other changes except to spend at least an hour and a half each evening at some physical activity.

He revisited me for an annual check-up recently. Never having been an athlete, he had started with walking and went on to jogging. Soon his wife was doing the same. The eyestrain was forgotten, his weight was down to normal, he looked and felt younger and reported that he slept better, worked more efficiently and enjoyed life more.

If all this sounds too simple, I assure you there are a great many like him.

What about eyestrain in children?

Providing there is no disease or need for glasses, the same explanations and remedies apply, only more so. The younger the child, the more physical activity he requires. There is more about this in Chapter 6 on children's eyes.

Do I harm my eyes by using them too much?

The answer is "No." Eyes don't wear out. You do **not** damage the eyes by excessive use even though there is discomfort from strain or fatigue. Most people fear blindness more than any other affliction. There are many elderly, retired persons who have nothing to do but read or watch television but who deny themselves such diversions in order to "save" their eyes — for fear they will "wear them out" and lose their sight. They are frightened by the symptoms of eyestrain which are natural with excessive use and which cause discomfort but no physical damage. They are frightened by the diminished sharpness of vision and by greater dependence on glasses (see Chapter 17) — but this is natural with advancing age and will occur whether the eyes are used constantly or not at all.

I often cite the example of the identical twin boys whose glasses were practically alike. When they grew up, one became a farmer who hardly ever had time to read, the other a proofreader who spent all his days reading fine print and his evenings poring over his stamp collections. By age seventy, both men were still wearing glasses with identical prescriptions and had equally healthy eyes.

The eyes are made to be used at all ages. With rare exceptions, as in certain diseases in which the ophthalmologist will recommend restraint, you need have no qualms about using your eyes as much as you wish. They won't deteriorate from use, no matter how much use they get. Barring accident or disease, the eyes will last a lifetime.

Happily, the same is true for people with only one functioning eye — where the other eye is useless. (See Chapter 10.)

Is there anything I can do to minimize eyestrain when excessive close work is unavoidable?

There is another category of eyestrain which simply cannot be avoided — the strain resulting from an overwhelming amount of concentrated and prolonged close work. One remedy under such conditions, which I discovered while in medical school, is merely a temporary subterfuge, used only under extreme fatigue, as when more study was necessary and it was already past 2 A.M. This consisted of alternate hot and cold compresses applied with a wrung-out towel to the closed eyelids for a total of four or five minutes. Physiologically this is quite sound — temporarily reducing fatigue by stimulating the circulation with sudden changes of temperature enabled us to study on for another hour or so. This is similar to the cold shower and rub-down between the halves of a football game.

For work done under excessive illumination or glare, I often recommend slightly tinted or polaroid glasses even if no prescription is required. Conversely where light in the working or reading area is too dim, simply increasing the illumination or placing it properly will help.

Wrongly placed light is a common cause of distress. A lamp or window **facing** the reader or worker reflects light from a shiny surface or a glossy page so that he is obliged to peer through the glare. This is especially true of student lamps which are wrongly placed at the front of the desk.

The remedy lies in placing the source of light on the side. For right-handed students, the light should be on the left side — otherwise the pen in the right hand casts a shadow on the page.

Should my glasses be safety glasses?

This question is now academic because by federal law all eye glasses must be safety glasses — either laminated glass, which may be somewhat thick and heavy, or specially treated (case-hardened) glass. A third choice, the plastic lens, is becoming more popular each year. Plastic is as safe as safety glass, very much lighter in weight, rarely becomes fogged by moisture, and corrects the focus practically as well as glass. It has one disadvantage: it scratches more easily than glass. You can avoid scratching or dulling of the surface of your plastic lenses by never laying them face down or polishing them. Instead, wash them in cold water, then gently pat (not wipe) them dry with a cloth or tissue. Always carry them in a case with a soft lining.

For other facts on safety glasses, see Chapter 8 on prevention of blindness from injury.

Do I need tinted glasses? Sun glasses?

Usually not — with a few exceptions. Sometimes I will prescribe slightly tinted lenses for patients with eye ailments which make them more sensitive to bright light, or for patients with very fair skin and light colored eyes. Such eyes have too little of their own protective iris pigment to screen out excessive light. I occasionally order slightly tinted lenses for patients who work under glaring illumination or on shiny surfaces. Use of excessively bright light over long periods will not damage the eyes of most normal persons though it is not advisable and can cause some fatigue and discomfort.

"Sun glasses" are darker than those just described. They are not necessary except for skiers, lifeguards or drivers who are exposed to excessive light for long periods. Most people quite rightly don't bother wearing sun glasses. The normal eye has its own device for automatically controlling the amount of light which enters: the pupil becomes smaller as the light becomes brighter.

A simple experiment will illustrate this dramatically. Stand before a mirror in dim light and look at your pupil. Switch on a flashlight so that the light falls on the eye. You will see the pupil promptly contract. This reduces the amount of light which enters the eye. We all know those who would not dream of being out in daylight without dark glasses. In most cases this is unnecessary and merely a matter of habit, but not at all harmful.

Some people who must wear glasses constantly have sun glasses made with their own prescription ground into them. This is often as much for cosmetic purposes as it is for comfort because it makes one appear not to be wearing "glasses" — merely attractive sunglasses. There is no harm in this.

There are now available chemically treated glasses which darken automatically in bright light and become clear indoors. They are mostly gadget and usually quite expensive. For the same price one can almost buy two ordinary pairs, one clear and one sun, and thus have the added advantage of a spare pair.

Can I become too dependent on glasses?

Not really. But dependence is a relative term. You may require lenses so strong that you are almost helpless without them. You could then justly be called dependent upon glasses, although it is still true that you do no damage by not wearing them — you merely do not see well.

The better the vision without glasses, the less likely you are to be dependent on glasses, but this varies with the individual's sensitivity and habit. Some hypersensitive, "perfectionist" persons with little optical defect are very uncomfortable without their glasses; conversely, there are casual, relaxed people with high degrees of error who do not bother with their glasses except when they need to see well. Habit, especially if established during formative years, is an important factor. I almost always encourage new wearers of glasses to use them only when they must, so that they retain the flexibility of being able to be comfortable without them.

I stress again: optically and medically it makes no difference to the health or preservation of the eyes whether glasses are worn constantly or rarely.

Is it possible to eliminate glasses by eye exercises?

Myths die hard. Many years ago an author named Bates published a book called "Perfect Sight Without Glasses" in which he advocated exercises to do away with the need for glasses. Many people still want to believe this but no one has ever proven scientifically that it is possible. If it did happen it was probably imaginary rather than real, more likely in people who wore glasses they never needed in the first place.

Why do some people squint when they don't wear their glasses?

To see better. Partly closing the lids (squinting) narrows the aperture through which light enters the eye and sharpens the focus — just as in photography one sharpens the picture by narrowing the diaphragm on the camera. A simple experiment will illustrate this: Blur your sight by removing your glasses. (If you don't need glasses, blur your sight by putting on the reading glasses of an older person.) Then look through a pinhole punched through a piece of heavy paper. This sharpens your sight in the same way squinting does.

Squinting is not harmful, merely unattractive. If it does not stop when proper glasses are worn, there may be some other reason for it and you should consult an eye specialist.

Why do some people need bifocals?

Some people, especially after the age of fifty, require different glasses for distance and for reading. They may have two separate pairs, or combine both into one. These are bifocals (bi = two). The upper part of the lens helps the eye to focus on distant objects, the lower part on near objects, such as print. There are also trifocals for people who need a third focus for middle distance, such as reading music. (For more about bifocals see Chapter 17.)

I have heard it said that I should 'change my glasses' once a year. Is that necessary?

Usually, no. With some exceptions. The exceptions are (1) in near-sighted children and (2) in many adults between the ages of forty-five and sixty-five. When growing children develop near-sightedness, it is common for that near-sightedness to increase a little with every inch of height. Thus, until they stop growing, their glasses become inadequate about once a year, sometimes oftener. After they have stopped growing, there is a leveling off and glasses need changing less frequently.

Many normal and most far-sighted people begin to need special glasses for reading around age forty-five. This is not caused by approaching blindness as many think, but by a natural loss of flexibility within the eyeball. (See Chapter 17 on abnormalities of focusing.) Such loss of flexibility may proceed with sufficient rapidity to require a change in reading glasses about once a year until age sixty-five, when the process usually levels off. Outside of these two age groups it is common for people to wear the same glasses for two, three or more years.

However, there is a far more important reason, unrelated to glasses, for you to be examined after age forty-five. You should be tested once a year for unsuspected glaucoma. (See Chapter 2 on glaucoma.)

What do you mean when you say 20/20, 20/40, or 20/70?

We use these terms to define sharpness of central vision. In most standard vision testing, you read the familiar Snellen eye chart at a distance of 20 feet. The upper number of the fraction expresses this distance, the lower one identifies the size letters you were able to read at 20 feet. Thus 20/70 vision means that you are able to read, at 20 feet (the upper number) only down to the line which a normal eye can read at 70 feet. 20/200 means that at the same 20 feet, you were only able to see the much larger letters a normal person can see at 200 feet. And 20/20 means seeing at 20 feet the line a normal eye can see at 20 feet, and is generally considered normal.

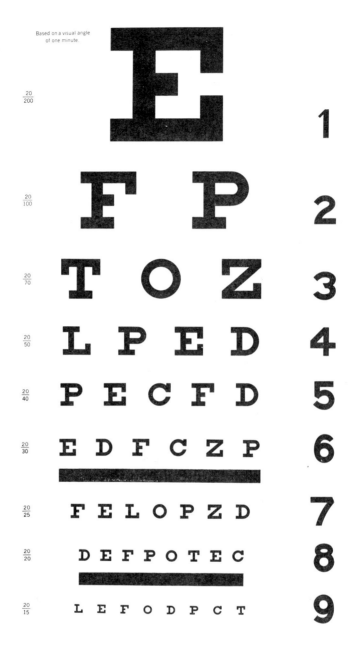

Fig. 1. This chart is only for illustration of how a vision chart looks. In order to use it for vision testing at a distance of 20 feet it would need to be enlarged about 3 times.

In some mass screening tests of vision, as in school and motor vehicle bureaus, this test is given by having you look into a machine which creates the same conditions optically. The results are roughly similar to those of the Snellen chart.

I am worried because I find I need my glasses much more as I get older.

This is no cause for alarm. As you age the focusing mechanism of the eye normally becomes less flexible. Therefore you are increasingly dependent on glasses to do the focusing for you.

Why do you sometimes use drops to examine for glasses?

Drops are used when required for greater accuracy in measuring far-sightedness or astigmatism or both, especially in young people. They are safe if I have first examined the eye and also checked the pressure to make sure there is no glaucoma.

Why are new glasses sometimes uncomfortable?

The most common reason is too much change at one time. This is most likely when you have had no examination for a few years. During that time your eyes may have changed a good deal, but so gradually that you were scarcely aware of it. Trying to give you three or four years worth of change all at once can be confusing. On such occasions I often prescribe a partial correction to be worn for six to twelve months, then the rest of the change next time. Such partial changes can thus be made with little or no discomfort.

Another cause of discomfort is switching from one type of lens to another. People being introduced to bifocals for the first time are occasionally uncomfortable. If you have worn bifocals before, you may be confused at first if the reading segments on your new ones are slightly different from the old in size, shape or position. If possible, it is better to show the optician your old bifocals so that he may match them in the new prescription.

The curvature of the new lenses can be a source of discomfort. It is possible to grind the same prescription correctly on different base curves. A patient accustomed to one set of base curves may find new ones uncomfortable at first, even though the strength of the lens is correct. This can sometimes be avoided if you make a point of showing your old glasses to the optician when you order your new prescription filled. (See Chapter 17.)

The new styles of oversized frames have given many people trouble, especially those whose glasses are strong and thick even in the old-style, conventional sized frames. Increasing the size of the lens means increasing its thickness and its weight and makes for greater difficulty in fitting the optical center of the lens precisely in front of the pupil. Failure to do this may lead to confusion, double vision or eyestrain — even if the frame is in the height of fashion, over-priced because it bears the name of a famous designer, and makes you look like an owl.

Lastly, there is always the possibility of human error in making the new lenses. This is rare because opticians are careful, but it can happen. If you have discomfort or are in doubt, it takes but a few minutes for me to check your glasses and make sure they are correctly ground as prescribed.

Can my eyes be examined for glasses by a machine?
Machines can expedite the refraction (the measurement of far-sightedness or near-sightedness or astigmatism) and so are merely devices for saving time. The various machines we use are not new. They are newer and faster versions of devices that have been in use for over a century.

The measurement, whether made without the machine or with it, is the less important part of the test. Much more important is the decision: how much of the measurement should go into the prescription for your particular glasses. This requires skill and judgement. It can be provided only by one who is a specialist by virtue of training and experience. The machine can only measure, it cannot think or make medical decisions.

Explain "near-sighted," "far-sighted," "astigmatism," "presbyopia."

More technical and precise explanations have been put into the last two chapters in order to keep the rest of the book easy to read. The following explanations are very much simplified:

A **near-sighted** eye sees near objects better than those at a distance. Someone who is near-sighted often needs no glasses for reading, but must wear them to bring distant objects into focus.

A **far-sighted** eye sees in the distance more easily than near, but can also see at close range because the lens within the eye is able to change focus. In youth this is possible because the lens is flexible. With age the lens loses its flexibility, making focusing at close range more and more difficult. This is why the average far-sighted person between age forty and fifty must first start holding print further away and then wear glasses to do the focusing which the lens within the eye is no longer flexible enough to do. This condition is called **presbyopia**. Later in life, such a person might also need glasses even for distance, but weaker ones than those he uses for reading.

In **astigmatism** the focus is distorted by a difference in curvature of the surface of the eyeball in different meridia. This may be corrected by an astigmatic glass specially shaped to compensate for these differences.

2
Glaucoma: Sneak Thief of Sight

Mr. Williams had been a chauffeur all his adult life. At fifty-five, he had worked for the same bank executive for seventeen years, without an accident. He was alert and in good health.

Recently he had an accident. A checkup at the motor vehicle bureau showed 20/20 vision in each eye with the glasses he had dutifully "changed" each year. Shortly thereafter, he was in another bad accident in which a child on a bicycle was killed.

I saw him for the first time after his latest accident. He read 20/20 with each eye. But I found a far advanced glaucoma in his right eye and early glaucoma in the left. This had never been detected because his yearly examinations had been merely for "change of glasses" and had not included a test for pressure in the eyes. Typical of glaucoma, the "side-vision" of his right eye was almost gone. The child he had killed was riding a bicycle to the right side of his car. He never saw the child until he had hit him!

There are thousands with glaucoma, like Mr. Williams, who are not aware of their defective vision.

What is glaucoma?

Glaucoma (oversimplified) is increased pressure of the fluids within the eyeball. Normally the clear fluid which fills the eyeball is maintained under gentle pressure. (To find out how the eye regulates this pressure, see Chapter 16.) When

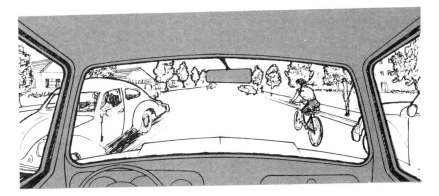

1. Normal. Side (peripheral) vision is unobstructed.

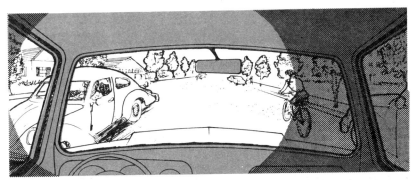

2. Side vision partly reduced by moderately advanced glaucoma. (The driver barely sees the child on the bicycle.)

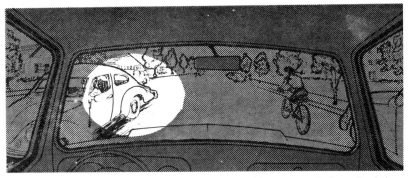

3. In late glaucoma there is practically no peripheral vision. This driver cannot see the child on the bicycle.

this regulating mechanism fails to work properly the pressure may rise, causing serious damage to the delicate structures within the eye. If the pressure is not reduced, these delicate structures may be destroyed, causing blindness.

Why is everybody afraid of glaucoma?

Glaucoma is one of the most dangerous of eye diseases and one of the most frequent causes of blindness — unnecessary blindness. Yet it is easy to prevent this blindness by controlling the glaucoma if it is detected early.

If it is easy to control why then is glaucoma so dangerous?

It is dangerous because in many instances it causes no pain and therefore gives no warning of its presence until it is too late. It is truly the thief of sight. Most other diseases are revealed by pain or other disturbance. A person suffering from glaucoma may not be aware of trouble until he has lost much of the sight in one eye and some of the sight in the other. This is not a rarity and has happened to many people.

Is it possible for me to lose part of my sight without knowing it?

Yes, because the pressure build-up is slow, the deterioration is gradual and painless, and the part of the vision lost is the "side" or the "peripheral" rather than the "straight-ahead" or the "central" vision.

If you lost your central vision, you would realize it immediately because you could not read or discern detail; but if you gradually lost your side vision you probably would not notice it. In glaucoma the central vision is usually retained until very late and you may think you are normal because you see well in the center and score 20/20 on the eye chart.

Is it possible for me to test my own side vision?

Yes, in a crude way, but doing so can do more harm than good. Only an ophthalmologist can test your side vision accurately enough to safely rule out glaucoma. It is easy for someone inexperienced to overlook defective side vision. You would then have a false sense of security about a very dangerous matter. Besides, by the time impaired side vision has become apparent, it is already late in the disease. You are far safer if you have your eyes and pressure checked each year if you are over forty, younger if there is glaucoma in your family of if you are quite near-sighted.

To get a rough idea of what extreme loss of side vision is like, try the experiment described on page 231. But bear in mind that any glaucoma patient who has reached the extreme state of "tubular" or "telescopic" vision there described cannot expect to have good peripheral vision restored.

Can vision lost from glaucoma ever be restored?

Unfortunately, treatment begun too late will not restore that portion of the sight already lost. The most one can expect from treatment is no further deterioration, but this too is questionable, because, in advanced cases where the loss has already been extensive, the deterioration may go on to complete blindness even after pressure has been made normal by medication or by surgery.

Is glaucoma contagious? Is it cancer?

Glaucoma is sometimes confused with a disease called trachoma because the names sound alike. Trachoma is a totally different and contagious eye disease rarely found in the Western world. Glaucoma is not contagious. It is not cancerous.

Is glaucoma related to high blood pressure?

It has no relation to blood pressure. People with high blood pressure need not have glaucoma; those with glaucoma may have normal blood pressure.

Who gets glaucoma? Does it run in families?

Anyone can have glaucoma. It is not common under the age of forty. Over forty, two out of every hundred normal men or women have the disease. The percentage gets higher at older ages and in those with glaucoma in the family. Not all children of parents with glaucoma have the disease. However, if you have glaucoma in your family you should have an annual checkup even before age forty.

Is it possible for me to recognize the symptoms of glaucoma?

Sometimes yes, occasionally no. In some people the symptoms are very severe. In some, there are no symptoms at all. In most, they are so slight that they may be overlooked unless you know what to look for.

Severe symptoms may begin with an acute attack of sudden blurring and severe pain, sometimes enough to cause nausea and vomiting. Such people are fortunate, in a sense, because the severity of the symptoms compels them to seek help quickly. (However, in some people the nausea and vomiting may be so severe that the blurring and ocular pain are not noticed and they mistakenly think they have a mere gastro-intestinal upset.) With prompt treatment of the glaucoma the sight is usually saved, but this must be begun within 24 hours. Speed is important. If pressure has not been relieved within 48 hours — by means of drops, internal medication, and, if necessary, emergency surgery — vision begins to deteriorate.

The most dangerous kind of glaucoma, by contrast, presents no symptoms at all — dangerous because even alert people may be unaware of trouble until, at their annual checkup, the ophthalmologist finds their eye pressure high. If such people have skipped one or more annual examinations, they could, in the interim, have lost considerable "side" vision without realizing it, and lost it irretrievably. The only protection against this kind of glaucoma is the annual eye examination.

The third group makes up the majority of glaucoma patients — those with symptoms which they **can** recognize if only they **know** what to look for.

What are these symptoms?
  Slightly oversimplified, they are:
  1. Disturbance in vision
  2. Discomfort
  3. Halos.

1. Visual Disturbance — usually foggy, misty or blurred vision, often intermittent rather than constant; usually slight but occasionally more severe. Glasses may repeatedly become inadequate and require too frequent changes. This symptom can be doubly misleading because after age forty many normal people experience difficulty in vision merely because of natural eye changes that come with age and require only glasses for correction. On the other hand, many with glaucoma have neglected it with disastrous results only because they thought all they needed was glasses.

2. Discomfort — pain in or around the eye, brow, forehead or head, usually on one side, usually slight but can be pronounced at times, and can be intermittent. There may be watering of the eyes or difficulty in adjusting to brightness or darkness. Again, there are other conditions which can cause such discomfort.

3. Halos — if they are present, halos are more typical

of glaucoma than are blurring or pain because few other conditions cause true halos. Halos should not be confused with "rays" which are normal and which can be made to radiate outward from a light by looking at the light through half shut eyes. A glaucoma halo is a true **circle surrounding** a light. It is seen best at night or in a dark room while looking at a small distant bright light. It is usually faint, white or colored, and may come and go.

You may have glaucoma with only one of the above symptoms but if **any two** or **all three** appear and disappear **together**, the probability is greater that glaucoma is present, and you should see an eye specialist.

Can people without glaucoma have these symptoms?

Yes. Not everyone with these symptoms has glaucoma. Many have other conditions. Only an eye specialist can decide whether or not they indicate glaucoma. The patient can only recognize the symptoms and report them to the eye specialist for his evaluation. If he does not have glaucoma, the ophthalmologist will tell him so.

How promptly should I see an eye specialist?

If it is an **acute** attack, with **severe** pain and/or blurring — you should get attention **very** promptly — within 24 hours.

If your symptoms (1, 2 and 3 above) are only mild and transient, your visit to the ophthalmologist need not necessarily be a "same-day" emergency. Neither should it be postponed for weeks if the doctor is booked far in advance. A phone call **describing your symptoms** to him or to an alert secretary will probably get you a "squeeze-in" appointment within a week or so, or you may be referred to another specialist who is less busy. If you call and get an answering service, find out what time you can call back and speak to his **office nurse personally**.

How do I find an eye specialist in such an emergency?

If you do not know an eye specialist, you can be referred to one by your family doctor, by your local hospital, or by the medical society of the county in which you live. (Now some Yellow Pages in telephone directories list them under "Ophthalmologists" or "Eye Specialists.") If it is not an emergency and you want to know more about qualifications and training of an eye specialist, see Chapter 15.

Does the examination hurt?

No. The specialist will examine your eyes and will do one or more tests for glaucoma depending on your history and on what he finds. If the results are doubtful or borderline, he may repeat the tests sometime later or do others known as "provocative" tests (so called because they "provoke" the glaucoma to show itself). All the tests, including the provocative tests, are entirely painless.

If the doctor finds glaucoma, what are my chances of saving or losing my eyesight?

If there is glaucoma, treatment begun early holds an excellent promise of success. The sight may be preserved for a great many years or a lifetime with little inconvenience beyond using eye drops a few times a day. There is no need to limit use of the eyes because of glaucoma.

Will I ever need an operation for glaucoma?

Most glaucoma patients do not need surgery. In a minority of patients drops alone may not control the disease and surgery may be required. An operation, if necessary, is very successful in the great majority of cases. The purpose of the operation is to preserve whatever vision you have left by minutely altering the structure of the eye to create a tiny safety valve which automatically reduces the pressure whenever it rises — just like the safety valve on the boiler or on the radiators in your home. It is usually done under local anesthesia and is painless. Failures or complications are a rarity. Most patients are out of bed next day, home in a few days, and back at work in a week or two. After the operation, the eye usually sees as well as it did before, and normal pressure is maintained with fewer drops or none at all.

If the operation is so easy and so often successful, why not operate on me now so that I don't need to bother with drops or worry about deteriorating vision?

That's a sensible question, and the answer in some cases might be "why not?" There are several reasons. Most important, we surgeons go on the principle that if conservative treatment is successful, don't operate. It's a matter of balancing risks: whether the small risk of deterioration in a chronic disease, carefully watched, is greater than the small risk of something going wrong during or after surgery. As you know, no operation is foolproof, no matter how well performed and no matter how favorable the statistics.

I always decide these questions by asking myself "What would I do if this patient were a member of my own family?" In such a case I would probably decide to avoid the risk of surgery — that is, unless I found the pressure going out of control or the peripheral vision deteriorating. As long as I could check the pressure and vision every few months, I would be conservative.

Of course, if you were going away to a remote part of the world for a year or more, as do some missionaries or Peace Corps workers, I would probably operate.

To sum up —

Glaucoma is an "all or none" disease. If discovered early, the cooperative patient can usually lead a normal life.

If discovered too late or neglected, it is a disaster.

The first and most important safeguard is the annual eye examination; the other is the patient's awareness of the possible danger signs of mild glaucoma so that he recognizes them if they appear and does not wait until next year's examination to consult his specialist.

If you don't have glaucoma, you may want to stop here. If you do have it, or want to know more, read on:

Other questions glaucoma patients often ask

What does the treatment of glaucoma consist of?

Before answering this question, I must remind you that the treatment of any eye disease is a highly specialized, highly sophisticated process which is learned only by many years of training. Glaucoma, like other such ailments, occurs in many variations and degrees. It is imperative that treatment (what kind, how much, how often, etc.) be meticulously tailored to the individual patient. What is right for another patient could be, literally, poison for you. Therefore, answers must necessarily be in generalities, and only your specialist can be more specific.

Generally speaking, all glaucoma treatment aims at reducing the high pressure within the eyeball to prevent pressure-damage to the delicate nerves. Failure to keep this pressure down results in gradual (often unnoticed until too late) destruction of these nerves and incurable reduction in sight.

The most common treatment consists of eye drops. Your ophthalmologist carefully determines the kind of drop, its strength, and the frequency of its use depending on all the factors in your individual case. Some patients require pills or capsules taken by mouth, in addition to drops or instead of them.

How important is it that my treatment be followed to the letter?

The faithfulness with which you follow instructions for the use of your medication may well determine whether or not your sight will be preserved. This does not mean that medicine to be used at a given time cannot be a half-hour late or early; it **does** mean that drops ordered five times daily should not be used only two or three times.

What if my drop seems to run out the instant I put it in?

It is important that the drop not only go into the eye but that it **stay** in. The drop is useless if it lands outside the eye or if it is instantly forced out by a quick squeeze of the eyelids. Drops are best administered when the patient learns to do it himself because he quickly becomes accustomed to his own manipulation and does not resist. As in anything else, practice is required.

What is the right way to put drops into my eyes?

The best way to take drops is while looking into a mirror. If your vision is poor, use a magnifying mirror. Wash your hands. Draw a small amount — a drop or two — out of the bottle with the eye dropper. (Do not fill the dropper because a full dropper squeezed into the eye wastes much expensive medication.) Hold the dropper lightly. With the forefinger of the other hand gently draw the lower lid down and away from the eye, creating a little space between the lid and the eyeball. Into this space, gently deposit a small drop out of the tip of the dropper (**anywhere** inside the lower lid, near the middle or near either corner). Now — and this is important — do **not** instantly let go of the lower lid because this will allow much of the drop to be squeezed out and wasted; instead continue to hold the lower lid lightly away from the eyeball for another five or ten seconds. This keeps the medicine in contact with the eyeball and helps its absorption into the eye. The drop is much more effective when taken this way.

I have tried using the mirror and it's too difficult.

Some patients prefer to instill their drops "by feel" rather than while looking into a mirror. This method is best used while the patient is lying down, face up, or sitting with the head bent backward. He then draws the lower lid away with one hand, and looks upward above his forehead to get the upper lid out of the way. With the other hand he holds the tip of the dropper close enough to the corner of the eye near the nose so that the drop falls into the eye. With this method, too, it is best to keep the lower lid drawn away from the eyeball for about ten seconds to give the drop a chance to spread over the eye and be absorbed.

Is there any harm in getting too much of the drops into my eye?

No. If you are not sure the drop has gone in or stayed in, do not hesitate to instill a second, or a third, or more until you are certain that one has stayed in. The space between the eye and the lid holds only one drop so no harm is done by an excess — it merely wastes the additional drops.

If I can't use drops, is there any way I can put the medicine into my eye?

Yes, there are two methods, both good, both with minor drawbacks, and both a little more expensive than the conventional eye drops.

One is a simple mechanical device which sprays a mist containing a measured amount of the prescribed medicine into the open eye. Some people who have great difficulty learning to instill conventional drops find this easier. Ask your eye specialist.

The other is a thin, wafer-like disc which contains a

measured amount of the prescribed medication. The disc is placed under the eyelid and allowed to remain there. Once inserted, the patient is scarcely aware of its presence. In the course of a number of days or a week the medicine is released to the eye at a very slow but uniform rate. This eliminates the need of putting drops into the eye at frequent intervals. Again, ask your specialist.

If I have prescriptions for more than one kind of drop does it matter which one I use first?

It rarely matters which is used first. But, where two **kinds** of eye drops are due at a given hour, it is best to allow at least three minutes between the first and the second.

Many eye drops today come in plastic squeeze-bottles which deliver only one or two drops at a time, eliminating the dropper. Some companies, despite my advice, still manufacture a bottle which is too stiff. This makes it difficult for older patients who have arthritis of the hands or whose hands tremble if they are obliged to squeeze hard to get a drop. They should ask their pharmacist to transfer the solution into a sterile conventional eye dropper bottle.

Do drops hurt or burn?

They may, slightly and for only a few minutes. Much depends on the strength of the drop and your own sensitivity. After you are used to the drops, there is little or no discomfort.

Do drops cause blurring?

Sometimes; and then only in the beginning. Some glaucoma drops make things look darker temporarily because they make the pupil smaller and so allow less light to enter the eye (like the under-exposed photograph when the lens opening is made too small). Strangely, the same small pupil may bring objects into better focus just as a small camera-lens opening results in a sharper picture.

Other kinds of glaucoma drops may cause temporary enlargement of the pupil. Either kind could produce a brief cramp-like sensation in the eye or brow, or transient redness.

May I use someone else's glaucoma drops if I run out of mine?

Never, never, unless you are absolutely sure that they are not merely glaucoma drops but the **very same** glaucoma drops as yours **and** you have verified this with your ophthalmologist. If you have spilled or run out of the drops it is better to delay until your druggist remakes them than to use another's. It is a good idea, especially if you travel, to have a spare bottle. Also, it is best **not** to wait until your bottle is empty before ordering a refill.

Should my drops be kept in the refrigerator?

Most glaucoma drops may be kept at room temperature. It is wise to avoid leaving eye drops above radiators, on window-sills where they bake in the sun or in automobiles parked in a hot sun. Some eye drops are best kept refrigerated and you will be so informed by the pharmacist. Traveling with such drops can be a problem. I instruct such patients to make a tiny refrigerator out of the smallest thermos jar. An ice cube put in with the tightly closed bottle of drops will keep the medicine cold for the trip.

Should I carry with me some information about my glaucoma in case of emergency?

Many glaucoma patients carry a "Glaucoma Identification Card" with their name, diagnosis, the kind, strength and frequency of their eye drops and the name of their eye specialist. This is handy to show another doctor such as an internist, or if you are unexpectedly admitted to a hospital.

Another advantage of such a card is that in an emergency it can explain the smallness of your pupils. Reason: most persons using glaucoma drops have small pupils; so do addicts using opium, heroin or morphine. A glaucoma identification card in your possession (or found on your person if you are injured or unconscious) can assure an emergency room doctor or a police officer, on seeing the smallness of your pupils, that you are not a drug addict, unconscious from an overdose.

```
                    GLAUCOMA IDENTIFICATION CARD
    Name: John Smith
    Address: 100 Central Ave., Lawrence, New York 11559
    Telephone: 516-CE9-0000

    Ophthalmologist:  Dr. Alan Jones     210 East 64 St., New York 10021
                                         212-TE8-0000

    Diagnosis: Chronic Open Angle Glaucoma R. Eye

    Medication: Pilocarpine 2% R. Eye every 4 hours
                Epifrin ½% R. Eye twice daily
                Diamox 125 mgm. every 8 hours

    If hospitalized, please see that the above patient obtains these medications.
                                                       Alan Jones, M.D.

    TO EMERGENCY ROOM DOCTOR          The constricted pupil is the result
    TO POLICE OFFICER                         of pilocarpine drops.
```

Fig. 3.   Sample Glaucoma Identification Card.

Does diet affect my glaucoma? Are there any rules to follow regarding diet, activity, etc.?

Very few. Patients with certain types of glaucoma should avoid **strong** coffee or tea, **large** quantities of water or other beverages taken at one time (no restriction on small amounts taken at intervals). There are no restrictions on use of the eyes, even to excess. However, people with some types of glaucoma should avoid total darkness such as in movie theaters (plays, or night sports under floodlights are permitted because darkness is not total). The total darkness of a bedroom is no problem because pressure tends to drop during sleep. However, in severe insomnia with long hours spent lying awake in the dark, it is best to have some light — or better still to read, which helps the insomnia, too.

None of these prohibitions may apply in your case. Ask your ophthalmologist.

Could my glaucoma medicine interfere with other medicines now taken by mouth? Could other medicines worsen my glaucoma?

Yes. Be sure to inform any doctor who prescribes medicine for you that you have glaucoma. In certain kinds of glaucoma, it is best to be cautious when taking medicines containing belladonna (or similar drugs) commonly used in stomach disturbances. Also if you are taking acetozolamide (Diamox or a similar substance) by mouth for your glaucoma, this substance is also a diuretic (a drug which improves the function of your kidneys). If your family doctor then prescribes another diuretic in addition, not knowing that you are taking one for the glaucoma, you may be getting more improvement in kidney function than you need.

A telephone conversation between your general doctor and your eye specialist can set such matters straight in a moment. Or, show him your glaucoma identification card, which will contain most of the information he needs.

Does glaucoma ever get better or get cured by itself?

Practically never, and most patients require drops as long as they live. Occasionally, after months or years of drops, pressure may remain low even after the drops are stopped for some time. This is rare and still requires the precaution of checkups at intervals determined by the ophthalmologist — because high pressures can recur.

3
Cataract

"Mrs. Jones, you will be relieved to hear that your failing vision is due to early cataract." This sounds flippant, even cruel. It is neither. I go on to explain to Mrs. Jones: "When you are past sixty or sixty-five you may develop one of a dozen eye diseases which accompany old age. Only one is curable. Fortunately for you, of all the diseases you could have had, you've picked the curable one — cataract."

In the following pages I have condensed the questions asked by thousands of cataract patients and their families and simplified the answers.

What is cataract?

Cataract is a clouding of the lens within the eyeball. The lens lies just behind the pupil. When it is clear, it helps to focus the eye so that objects are seen sharply. In many older people this lens becomes slowly and progressively cloudy. This is cataract. In ancient times it was thought that water, falling down over the pupil, made it white and opaque. (Waterfall = cataract: hence the name.)

What are the symptoms of cataract?

Blurring or clouding of vision, slight at first, often beginning in only one eye. Some people may see multiple images or experience glare in bright light. The cloudy lens creates this glare by scattering light rays just as dust on a windshield causes dazzling by scattering the bright light of an oncoming headlight. This is partly relieved by wearing sunglasses.

Caution: All the symptoms mentioned above could also be from other eye conditions. Only your eye specialist can determine the cause. There is an even better reason for consulting him: If the diagnosis is cataract, an **early** examination is desirable because later on, the more advanced cataract will make it more difficult for him to look into the pupil and examine the back of the eye. Thus, other diseases which might also impair the vision would not be discovered until after removal of the cataract.

I always thought cataract was a 'skin' over the eye and that it had to be peeled off.

A cataract is not a 'skin' over the eye. It is not 'peeled off.' The opaque lens is behind the pupil, not in front of it. It is removed from within the eye by a delicate but painless operation.

You mean I need an operation?

Yes, but not now, because your cataracts are not yet far enough advanced and your sight is still sufficient for your needs. Most cataracts progress slowly, gradually making the vision poorer. When you see this happening, don't worry because it is normal and expected. The more cloudy your vision becomes, the nearer you are to having your cataracts removed and your sight restored — usually completely restored.

How long will it be before my eye is ready for an operation?

There is no way to predict. Some cataracts develop more slowly than others. Yours could take a few months or many years. Some cataracts progress only a little, then stop. If so, you may never require surgery.

How bad does it have to get? Must I become blind before you operate?

No. While a more advanced cataract is a little easier to remove, we need not wait for it to be fully ripe (completely opaque). Our methods are so improved that we can operate whenever you find your sight too poor for the kind of work you do. I have removed early cataracts from a jeweler as young as fifty-four who had 20/40 vision, good enough to drive a car, but too blurred for his kind of work. On the other hand, I have been able to dissuade from operation many older patients who do not work or drive, who care little about reading or television and who are quite comfortable with partly reduced sight.

Is age important? Won't I be too old for an operation?

No. In fact, age is an advantage. I would rather operate on you in your eighties or nineties than in your sixties because the older you are, the more easily your cataract comes off (provided, of course, that you have not waited so long that it has become **over**-ripe). One of the nice things about this operation is that it is usually done under local anesthesia. We dislike putting elderly patients to sleep with a general anesthetic unless we must. Local anesthesia is easy, safe and painless at any age. However, if your surgeon advises a general anesthetic in your particular case, he undoubtedly knows it would be better.

My oldest and most grateful patient is a highly literate and alert little lady of ninety-seven who was blind until I removed her cataracts five years ago. She now has 20/30 vision and, because of her other infirmities, spends all her days and much of her nights reading. This is not an isolated instance; most of my colleagues have similar patients.

Do I need to stop reading because I am developing cataract?

Not in the least. You may read, sew, watch television or use your eyes in any way you please. Use or non-use of the eyes has no effect whatever on the progress of a cataract. Nothing you do or don't do will change its course one bit.

Must one be old to have cataract?

No, cataracts can occur at any age although by far the greatest number are found in older people. The technical term for this is "senile" cataract, to distinguish it from other kinds of cataract such as congenital, juvenile, traumatic, secondary, etc. I never use the term "senile" (except in scientific writing) because it refers only to chronological age. I have known too many patients in their eighties and nineties who are mentally alert and anything but senile, although I had removed their "senile" cataracts twenty years earlier.

What are the other kinds of cataract besides 'senile'?

Fortunately they are rare, but cataracts can form in young people and are sometimes found at birth, especially if the mother of the newborn had had German measles during her pregnancy.

People with diabetes are a little more likely to develop cataract at an earlier age. The same is true of those with glaucoma, even if the pressure is controlled.

Injury to the eye can cause cataract at any age as can certain diseases of the interior of the eye.

Radiation can result in cataract. The effect of X-Rays is well known and accounts for the elaborate precautions that are taken to protect the eyes from them. Ultraviolet rays do not penetrate the eyes deeply enough to reach the lens; their action is superficial, as in snow blindness, sunburn, or sunlamps. But infra-red rays do penetrate and cause cataracts, as in the case of glass-blowers, and stokers of olden times.

Modern times have brought other hazards or potential

hazards. While not yet proven, there is now some suspicion that excessive exposure to short-wave radiation such as radar apparatus, microwave ovens and even improperly constructed television sets may have adverse effects on the eye. We hope to have more definite information from the government on this subject in the near future. Meanwhile it would be wise to sit at least six feet away from television sets, especially color TV, and to make as certain as possible that microwave ovens do not leak and that they are tightly closed if you use them at all.

How is it that more people are having cataract operations than years ago?
Because cataracts are more common in older persons and because the population has increased with people living to an older age. In addition, with improvement in surgical technique and instruments, a very high proportion of cataract operations results in perfect vision. This induces more people to have the operation performed.

Is it possible to prevent 'senile' cataract?
Because the exact cause of cataract is unknown there is as yet no way of preventing it. Much research is now being done on this subject.
Meanwhile we can only say that 'senile' cataract usually accompanies age, without being able to explain why many older people do **not** suffer from it.

My daughter just told me that you informed her three years ago that I was developing early cataract. Why didn't you tell me?
In the early stages of cataract I often do not inform the patient because many of these cataracts progress little or not at all over the years. Had I disclosed this to you it would

have been a source of needless anxiety for the past three years.

Now that your sight is poorer, I feel that you would be more frightened **not** knowing what makes it so, than knowing about it and being assured that it is curable.

Although my vision is cloudier, how is it I can now read without my glasses?

This sometimes happens in early cataract, and it is called "second sight." Slight optical changes in the clouding lens make it more near-sighted, enabling you to see quite well at close range without the glasses you formerly had to wear.

Can't you give me stronger glasses to see better?

Stronger glasses will not help. Your trouble is not that your glasses are too weak but that your pupil is cloudy and will remain cloudy no matter how strong or how clear a lens you place before the eye. It is as though you had a badly smeared window and you tried to see better through it by lowering a perfectly clean window in front of the cloudy one.

Must the eye be removed from its socket for operation and then put back?

No. This is a common superstition, totally untrue.

Is the operation difficult?

No. For an operation which is just about the most delicate in all surgery, it is surprisingly easy — for the patient as well as for the skilled surgeon.

Do you operate on both eyes at the same time?

No. It is possible but in most cases it is better not to. Usually one eye ripens ahead of the other. But I have on occasion operated on both cataracts a few days or a week apart, when both eyes were in an advanced stage of readiness.

Can my cataract be completely cured?
Yes, in most cases completely cured.

What do you mean by "most cases"?
There is no operation in the world which is successful 100 times out of 100. Unlike building a bridge or a machine out of inert materials whose strengths can be known in advance, surgery on living tissue often encounters unknown factors beyond the control of the patient, the surgeon or the hospital. Despite all the elaborate tests we do and the precautions we take, there is always the remote chance of something not going according to plan. The only honest answer I can give you is a statistical one: I have performed over 6000 cataract operations; more than 95% resulted in normal vision — 20/20, 20/30 or 20/40.

When you say normal vision, do you mean without glasses?
No, with cataract glasses. Either spectacles or contact lenses.

You mean contact lenses which are really cataract glasses?
Precisely. Most of my cataract patients prefer contact lenses after I have operated on them, and they love them — unless they are too feeble, old or unsteady to insert them themselves. Once they have used them, they much prefer them to spectacles.

Why do I have to wear a cataract glass at all?
Because when I operate to remove the cataract from within the eye, I am really removing the clouded lens. Therefore, you must wear a lens of the same strength to take

its place, either in the form of spectacles or contact lenses. Without the glass the eye will see, but will not focus clearly.

Is there a new kind of cataract lens which is put inside the eyeball?

Yes there is. It is called an intraocular lens (intra = inside). It is put inside the eye by the surgeon at the time he removes the cataractous lens. It may also be inserted at a later time but this requires a separate operation. It is very tiny, almost weightless and is made of a plastic material which is supposed to have no harmful effect on the delicate interior of the eyeball.

The great advantage of the intraocular lens is that, by taking the place of the cloudy natural lens, it can focus the eye without the need of a cataract spectacle or contact lens. Of course, you will still require glasses for reading.

Its disadvantage is the possibility that the lens may not be tolerated and have to be removed. Although unlikely, such an occurrence would require another operation which could further damage the eye.

The intraocular lens is no longer in the primitive stage. Many thousands have been inserted in various clinics throughout the world with very few catastrophes. Yet many surgeons are a bit conservative and skeptical about using it, preferring to wait until more people have been subjected to this procedure without harmful results.

There is another reason why some of us are not in a hurry to use the intraocular lens. It is probable that within a few years a "continuous-wear" contact lens may become available (see Chapter 13 on contact lenses). This will probably be almost as effective as an intraocular lens and safer.

Is there any risk in not having the operation?

Not really, unless you develop pressure in the eye or

unless the cataract becomes over-ripe — it becomes liquefied, excessively soft and may disintegrate. Should that occur, you then have no choice but to operate. The chance of this is slight and I will check your eyes every few months to make sure it is not happening. Meanwhile, if you do not mind getting about with reduced vision, there is no harm or danger in waiting. Of course, your poorer sight makes you more prone to accident. But before that stage is reached, you will probably come and ask to have your cataracts removed.

If I have cataract in only one eye and good sight in the other, does the cataract have to be removed?

No, not as long as the cataract eye does not become over-ripe or develop glaucoma. Most one-eyed patients get along quite well (see Chapter 10). If the cataract becomes quite opaque or if you notice the second eye beginning to cloud, then operation on the first eye should be performed. Some patients never develop a cataract in the second eye.

However, those with occupations requiring **both** eyes working together should have the single cataract removed even though the opposite eye is clear. They then wear a contact lens over the operated eye.

The cataract operation on my first eye was very successful and I now have perfect sight with it. Why should I bother having the cataract on the second eye removed?

There are several reasons. Two good eyes see better than one. Also at your age the successfully operated eye could develop other diseases not related to the cataract. If you then have the second eye in reserve you are far less handicapped.

Most important of all, there is a possibility that the cataract in the second eye could become over-ripe. This can be a serious complication and could lead to pain, glaucoma and even the removal of the eye. I have seen this happen in patients who are so well satisfied with the first eye that they were willing to ignore the second until it was too late.

I have heard about a new machine and a new method to make the operation quicker and the convalescence shorter.

There are not one but several new machines and about twenty methods for removing cataracts. They are all about 95% successful, and those of us who do cataract surgery are constantly modifying and improving them.

A quick operation and a short convalescence do not necessarily mean a better result or one less prone to complications. Compared to the importance of good sight for the rest of your life, it matters little whether the operation takes fifteen or thirty minutes or whether you leave the hospital in one day or four.

Practically all good eye surgeons, using the method which in their experience has proven best and safest, obtain excellent results.

What do you mean by 'good' eye surgeons?

How to evaluate ophthalmologists and pick a good one, especially when contemplating surgery, is properly a matter of concern. I have therefore devoted a separate brief chapter to this subject. (See Chapter 15.)

This is about as much as most people want to know about cataract. A look at the diagram in the last chapter will clarify the subject further.

However, if you are more curious or if you have cataract, read on:

Are cataract lenses those very thick glasses?

They are heavier than ordinary spectacles. However, today they are thinner and lighter than formerly because they are specially designed and made of plastic rather than glass. Contact lenses, on the contrary, are almost invisible and almost weightless.

Which are better — cataract glasses or cataract contact lenses?

If I ever have cataracts, I would prefer, after operation, to wear contact lenses. Although your operation restores good sight with either kind of lens, there are two minor disadvantages to the cataract spectacle:

1. The glass makes objects look larger and closer than they really are. The contact lens gives more natural vision. This is because the contact lens is closer to the eye (in fact, in "contact" with the cornea) while the glass must be worn about a half-inch away from it.

To illustrate the magnifying effect of such a distance, take an ordinary magnifying glass and lay it on a printed page. There is practically no magnification because the glass is in "contact" with the page. Now move the glass a half inch away from the page and you will observe that the print becomes slightly enlarged.

2. The glass is perfectly focused only near the center — the sight through the rest of the lens is slightly distorted, so that the "side" vision ("peripheral" vision) is sometimes a little impaired. This is not true of the contact lens because, being in contact with the eyeball, it moves with the eye.

However, there are many thousands of people who have become accustomed to cataract spectacles and wear them quite comfortably, getting about and doing everything as they did before they developed cataracts.

Does the operation take long?

No. The actual removal of the cataract takes only a

short time. What keeps you on the operating table longer is the preliminary procedure and a series of elaborate precautions to make as certain as possible that everything goes well and painlessly.

You mean I will feel nothing?

You will feel me touching your face and eyelids but because of the local anesthetic you will feel no pain whatever. You may recall that as part of your regular examination I placed an instrument (tonometer) on your eyeball for a routine glaucoma test. You felt nothing, yet this instrument was in contact with your eyeball. The reason you did not feel it was because a minute earlier the nurse gave you a drop of local anesthetic. Without this drop you could not have tolerated even the touch of the instrument. Before I begin the operation, I will put the same kind of drops into your eye and you will feel no more than you did in the examination. Also, to prevent you from blinking while I work, I will inject a bit of anesthetic near the eyelids. With this, you feel no more than a momentary pinprick.

I have made it a practice in my office to introduce people with cataract to those already cured. There are usually one or two in the waiting room. To hear at first hand, from one who has just been through it, that the operation is painless and successful, is far more reassuring than anything I can say. As a result, patients whose surgery can be deferred do not spend months or years in dread of the prospect; those scheduled for early surgery enter the operating room almost casually, completely relaxed and confident — and thus make the operation even easier because they are not tense. In fact, having had a mild routine sedative before coming to the operating room, they usually fall into a quiet, natural sleep on the operating table before the operation is half over.

How can I prevent my friends and my employer from knowing that I will have cataract operations?

Simply by not telling them about your cataracts or about your prospective operation. Privacy is your privilege. You are wise to keep this to yourself and your family if you are sensitive about it for social or other reasons.

The great majority of my younger cataract patients, especially those who hold jobs, wear contact lenses which are invisible and reveal nothing about their operation.

I often operate on people in public life — including fellow doctors, surgeons and eye surgeons. Even though they and I know that their resulting vision will be 20/20 and that they will be able to function normally after operation, they are naturally concerned that their own patients will doubt their competence when word gets around that they have undergone cataract surgery. In such cases I advise them beforehand against making the matter public. Their hospital stay is short enough to minimize exposure. If that is not safeguard enough, I refer them to my former students in other cities. They get as good a job as I would have done and are back at work in two or three weeks, having been merely "out of town."

I had a heart attack three years ago and my activities are now limited. Will that interfere with my cataract operation?

Not necessarily. You can still have the operation because you don't require a **general** anesthetic. Neither the local anesthetic nor the operation itself is a strain on your system. Even a prolonged stay in bed, which doctors try to avoid in older people, is unnecessary. You are out of bed and sitting in a chair the day after operation.

Does my general health affect my cataract operation?

Of course, any chronic illness should be controlled as

well as possible before you enter the hospital. This is particularly true of such ailments as diabetes, high blood pressure, anemia, gout and any of the infections of the teeth, sinuses, chest, etc.

You will visit your family doctor or internist now and a week before you enter the hospital. I will telephone him to discuss your medical status. Also, he will check you when you have entered the hospital and he will be available to re-visit you there in the unlikely event that any new medical condition appears.

Should you develop any illness or even a cold before you are to enter the hospital, your operation would best be postponed — since there is rarely any hurry about a cataract operation. But, in that case, be sure to telephone me at once so that I may give your reservation to another patient on the waiting list.

How long will I be incapacitated after surgery?

Time varies considerably, depending on your individual case and on the techniques and precautions observed for your safety. As a rule, you sit up out of bed the day after operation, usually with only the operated eye covered by a light cotton patch and an aluminum eye shield. Most people go home between the second and sixth post-operative days. Remain fairly quiet at home for a week if your occupation is light or sedentary, three weeks if it is more active. Spend as little time in bed as possible. During that time the unoperated eye may be used, wearing the old glasses.

What restrictions are there on my activity during my convalescence?

For the first few weeks you will avoid heavy lifting, vigorous bending or exercise, and straining during bowel movements (use mild laxatives if necessary). When at home it would be better if you could avoid housework such as cleaning or bedmaking for a week or two, but you may prepare a light meal or wash a few dishes, or walk stairs carefully. You may need drops or salve in your eye one or more times daily; I prefer that you do not do this yourself but that someone at home do it for you. If everyone is away at work, you can still be given your medication three times a day: on arising, after working hours and at bedtime.

For the technique of instilling eye drops, see the chapter on glaucoma (Chapter 2).

When at home, you no longer need the cotton patch but you may continue to wear the light, perforated aluminum shield either constantly or only for sleep. This is merely a device for keeping the fingers out, not for keeping the eye closed. Once the patch has been discarded, it is much better for the operated eye to remain naturally open even if the shield is in front of it. Do not keep the lids tightly shut under the shield because you think you are protecting the eye. This is uncomfortable and actually delays the healing.

It is natural for an operated eye to be slightly red for a few weeks and this should be no cause for alarm. An occasional scratchy sensation can also be expected and diminishes in time. Itching can be annoying. One popular notion, which happens to be true, is that itching is a sign of healing. This is your only consolation for not being allowed to scratch or rub the eye — the shield is worn to prevent your doing that.

Excessive sensitivity to light is often experienced — understandably because the former cataract kept most light out of the eye. Now, with the pupil clear again, the eye is flooded with too much light. Dark glasses during the day are in order and will obviate the need to keep window shades down, especially if your home is sunny.

Sometimes you may notice that objects seen with the operated eye are colored blue or red. This is not abnormal and will gradually disappear.

How soon after operation will I get my glasses?

That varies a great deal depending on your sensitivity, the kind of operation performed, the amount of sight present in the other eye, etc.

Sometimes I let the patient wear a temporary lens in the center of the aluminum eye shield while he is in the hospital. This is done if there is no sight in the opposite eye or if the patient needs a constant demonstration of his newly regained sight for reassurance.

The temporary lens is usually only approximate — it does not attempt to focus the eye perfectly. There are several reasons for this. Most patients would be uncomfortable if an eye only recently blind were suddenly focused sharply. Also, during the first few weeks or months post-operative, the focus keeps changing as the eye heals more firmly. Keeping up with these changes would require a new cataract glass every two weeks or so. The cost would be prohibitive because such lenses are very expensive. There is no harm, and in fact a slight advantage, in delaying the permanent, perfect lens a few weeks or months. If the final lens is to be a contact lens, we usually wait two months.

During the entire post-operative period there is no objection to wearing your **old** glasses if they help the sight of your other eye. Dark glasses or dark clip-on glasses on top of your regular glasses may be more comfortable. Glasses may be worn over the aluminum shield even if they do not sit very well.

I have a friend who has had a cataract operation on one eye and sees well, but can't wear her glasses.

This is quite common with cataract spectacles but less so with contact lenses. There are good reasons for this, and your surgeon will explain them to you carefully before he operates on your first eye.

You will recall that a cataract lens, while it brings your

eye into focus (in place of the lens that was in your eye), also makes objects look larger, nearer and rounder. Now, if I were to put such a lens before your operated eye **combined with** an ordinary lens before the **other** eye, you could see two kinds of image — one large, the other normal. You would not tolerate this because you would not be able to "fuse" the two different sized images into one. This would lead to very annoying double vision.

With a contact lens the problem of double vision does not exist. There is little magnification since this lens is worn in "contact" with the eye — unlike the spectacle lens which magnifies because there is a space between it and the eye.

If you cannot or will not wear a contact lens, you may start off with "practice" cataract spectacles. On these, the unoperated eye is blocked by an opaque disc, forcing the operated eye to focus through the corrective lens. You will wear these glasses for practice only, i.e., limiting yourself to television (distance) and reading (near), and this only while sitting in a chair. Walking with this device comes later. You must remember that for months or years before operation your cataractous eye had not been used. Learning to focus this newly restored eye through a cataract lens will take patience and practice.

After the second eye is operated upon, the problem of making the two eyes work together hardly ever persists, because you will have already learned to focus with your first eye and you now have **two** cataract lenses **alike** instead of one cataract lens and one ordinary lens.

I repeat — with most patients such problems do not arise if they wear a cataract **contact** lens.

Why is it impossible to predict with certainty, before I have my operation, whether the result will be good or poor?

That is a very important question and all eye surgeons

prefer to answer it **before** they operate. So read this carefully:

Statistically the great majority of cataract operations (at least 95%) result in restoration of normal vision (20/20 to 20/40) or as good vision as ever existed before the cataract developed. Naturally, if an eye, for some other reason, has had poor vision earlier in life, one cannot expect removal of a cataract to make it **better** than it was before, only as good.

But I am not interested in statistics. I want to know what is going to happen to me. What about the few whose operations do not result in good vision?

There are several possible reasons:

First, as I explained earlier, any operation which deals with living tissue cannot be as predictable as a mechanical procedure such as building a bridge or a motor.

Second, the unforeseen such as hemorrhage or infection or poor healing is always a remote possibility despite the elaborate precautions taken by the surgeon and the hospital.

Third, the surgeon cannot be sure, before operation, that the rest of the eye is healthy. This is particularly true of the retina, that delicate structure at the back of the eye which receives the image after the clarity of the pupil is restored by the operation. It takes more than a perfect pupil to see well. The retina must also be in working order. But, before operation the doctor cannot see the retina because the cataract is in the way. Just as your cataract prevents you from seeing **out** of the eye, so it prevents the doctor from seeing **into** the eye. Thus both patient and surgeon are occasionally disappointed when, despite successful restoration of a beautifully clear pupil, the sight does not return to normal.

Fourth, it can happen that, after a successful operation, other conditions may develop later which are in no way related to the operation. Patients over sixty-five are prone to ailments such as poor circulation, hemorrhage, or retinal disease, even if they have never had a cataract or an operation. The uninformed patient quite naturally, but wrongly, attributes such mishaps to any operation performed recently or in the remote past.

However, it must again be stressed that for the overwhelming majority, the restoration of sight by cataract operation is a thrilling experience. This is equally true for the surgeon although he has performed the same operation thousands of times. Most patients are delighted to be able to go back to the work or the hobby that had been curtailed by their poor vision. A few make fresh starts in new fields of endeavor. I recall two of my post-operative patients whom I saw again recently:

H.B., an eighty-two year old retired electrical engineer, formerly blind, now with 20/20 vision. After his sight was restored, he taught himself wire sculpture. Now eighty-five, he exhibits his works and sells them. He has also taught the art to the other members of his Golden Age Club and they are all very busy making and selling wire sculptures.

B.P., an eighty-six year old retired iceman, healthy and vigorous, had been blind at eighty. After cataract operations at age eighty-three, his vision was normal. On a recent re-visit, his wife who accompanied him asked me to put the cataracts back into his eyes! Reason: "Now that he can see again he's running after other women!"

In no way should this be construed as recommending cataract operation for restoring any function other than sight! It does show that it is never too late for a new start.

4
Detachment of the Retina

Retinal detachment used to mean blindness. Today most detachments can be cured. This gratifying and spectacular improvement in outlook has taken place — not over a few centuries — but in the space of forty years. In the 1930's, an eye with retinal detachment was almost certain to remain blind. Fewer than one percent could be cured. Now, after years of research, surgeons, using modern discoveries in physics and engineering, can cure over 95% of detachments. Better still, we can now **prevent** detachment before it happens by a procedure so simple and painless that it is sometimes done in the office or in the clinic, without anesthesia, without surgery, and without the need for admission to the hospital. More about all this at the end of the chapter.

What is retinal detachment?

It is a separation of the retina from its normal position at the back of the eye. The retina is the innermost lining of the eyeball. It is the very delicate membrane which receives the focused image entering the pupil. The retina has been compared to the film which lines the back of the camera. It has also been compared to wallpaper lining the interior of a room, but this is inaccurate because wallpaper is firmly pasted to the wall over its entire extent, while the adherence of the retina to the inside wall of the eye is far from firm. In fact, it is physically attached to the inside of the eye in only two places: at the very back (the optic nerve) and at its front edge (the ciliary body). The rest of the retina, about 98% of it, is held in position by the gentle pressure of the eye fluids. Any part of the retina may detach.

What causes retinal detachment?

Imagine a tiny, fragile balloon which is kept in the shape of a sphere by being filled with fluid. Make a tiny hole in it and the fluid seeps out, causing it to collapse. This, in a way, is what happens when the retina tears and detaches.

A hole or tear ('tear' here refers to a torn retina; not to tear drops) may develop in any part of the retina but is most frequent near its front edge where it is thinnest. A spot which has been weak for years suddenly gives way. Nobody can predict when this will occur. It may be spontaneous, for no apparent reason, or it may follow a blow to the eye or to the head, or a bad jolt as in a fall or in an accident. Prize fighters are prone to detachment because of the frequent blows and jolts they receive. In susceptible persons, a tear may occur after violent coughing, sneezing, retching, straining at stool, heavy lifting or other physical exertion. In older persons, weakening of the structures or traction of a shrinking vitreous fluid may cause a tear. A near-sighted eye is a little more likely to have a tear because it is elongated and the retina is a bit "stretched."

By far the greatest number of people who are susceptible in this way never develop a tear. But where a tear does occur, some of the vitreous fluid leaks through and seeps behind the retina, causing it to move forward, away from the back of the eye. This further enlarges the tear, allowing still more seepage and a gradual increase in the detachment. (See the illustration on the opposite page.)

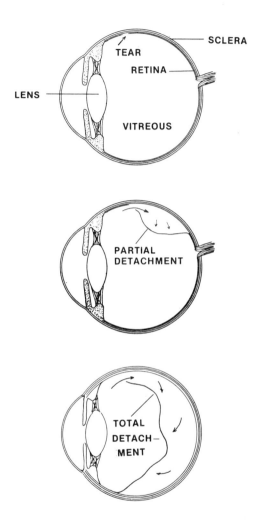

Fig. 4. Three stages of retinal detachment.

How do you know you have a detachment?

Sometimes you don't until it is moderately advanced. You yourself cannot see the retina because it is inside the eyeball, behind the pupil. It can be seen only by looking through the pupil with an ophthalmoscope. Your own first awareness may be a blur in part of your peripheral field of vision. The blur may be quite definite and is usually described by the patient as a shadowy area or "curtain" in one portion of the visual field which he tries to brush away but cannot, and which stays in the same position, moving only with movement of the eye.

This "curtain" is not the same as "spots" or translucent "threads" which are often present **without** detachment in many normal eyes, especially after age forty-five. Such spots or threads are caused by alterations in the vitreous or in the circulation of the eye — changes which are normal for that age.

But beware! Such spots could **also** be an early symptom of impending detachment, especially if they are accompanied by flashes. The patient has no way of determining whether his spots and flashes are a harmless variant or the sign of early detachment. Although the chances of the latter are about one in twenty, he should, if they persist more than a day or so, consult an eye specialist. This is all the more true if the symptoms occur a few days or weeks after a blow to the eye or head. The specialist dilates the pupils with drops and by means of a special magnifying ophthalmoscope examines all of the retina — an entirely safe and painless procedure.

Should a detachment be treated immediately?

If a detachment is found, it calls for reattachment without much delay because, by its very nature, it tends to increase. The longer a detachment lasts, the larger it becomes, the more extensive is the surgery required to reattach it, and the greater the chance of permanent residual defect in vision. If examination discloses only an early hole without detachment, you are lucky because a quick and permanent cure may be achieved by the use of a light beam, or a laser beam, or surface freezing, without actual surgery.

Even if there is no detachment or tear, the ophthalmologist still may find an area at the edge (periphery) of the retina which looks thin, as though it might tear eventually. He may advise no treatment but ask you to return for observation of the area at intervals and resort to the laser or freezing if the condition seems to be progressing toward a tear. This may prevent a detachment. He may also employ such a precautionary measure on your second eye if you have already had a detachment on the other one.

How is retinal detachment treated?

Reduced to its simplest terms, the goal of treatment for detachment of the retina is to return it to its normal position so that vision is restored and remains restored. An eye with a detached retina is about as useful as a camera with its film torn and hanging loose.

A spectacular example of progress in surgery

As recently as 1932, the eye with detachment was almost always doomed to blindness. In rare instances, if surgery was attempted, it was crude and heroic. It consisted of cutting a small hole in the back of the eyeball (the sclera) through which the surgeon briefly inserted a tiny stick of powerful chemical (potassium hydroxide) as close as possible to the estimated site of the detachment and the tear which caused it. Hopefully, the resulting severe chemical burn would cause sufficient scar inside the eyeball to seal off the tear and reattach the retina. (Sometimes this burn was so severe that it destroyed the eye.) The patient was confined to bed motionless for three pain-filled weeks. Successes were so rare that the operation was hardly ever performed except in desperation, as when an only remaining eye developed detachment.

Spot-welding

The breakthrough occurred when it became possible, after extensive experiments on animal eyes, to use tiny electrodes, 1/16 of an inch long, to apply high-frequency electric current to pin-point areas on the sclera just above the torn and detached retina. These applications created minute burns, ever so much finer, more delicate, more controlled and better aimed than did the single stick of potassium hydroxide. The eye barely became inflamed, pain was very slight, but the minute scars caused by these tiny burns acted as spot-welds to hold the retina in place, adherent to the choroid and sclera. No hole had to be cut because it was found, with more animal experiments, that a slight alteration in current allowed the electrode to make its own pinhole.

Immediately the cure rate went from less than 1% to better than 50%! In a few years, with further refinement in technique, it rose to 75%. Cures of retinal detachment became commonplace. Patients were no longer faced with almost certain blindness. Eye surgeons were elated.

Buckling

However, in one-fourth of the cases the operation was still a failure, or if successful, the detachment recurred later. After a great deal more animal experimentation, it was found that in certain cases it was not enough to bring the retina back to its normal position. With the retina a little too short for the slightly stretched eyeball, it might not hold firm, or if it did, it would detach again.

A still more delicate technique was then devised for shortening the eyeball to accommodate the shortened retina. At first, the procedure consisted of removing a tiny sliver of sclera and sewing the two edges together. Later, the technique was refined by taking a fold in the sclera, much as one would shorten a sleeve by tucking it. Still later, it was found possible to buckle the sclera to meet the retina, making it easier to gain adhesion for reattachment. To achieve this, bits of silicone — synthetic rubbery pellets or tubes — were implanted to change the shape of the eyeball so that the retina would stay reattached more securely.

Laser

After more years of research and animal experiments, another improvement supplemented the high frequency electrodes. It was found that a very high powered, highly concentrated and carefully aimed light beam could produce fine retinal burns to create the adhesions. From this, it was but a step to using laser beams for the same purpose, and these could be even more finely focused and more accurately aimed. Both the light beam and the laser beam have a great advantage: they can be "shot" into the eye from in front, through a dilated pupil, directly at the affected part of the retina under the clear (magnified) view of the surgeon, without any cutting, with no need to expose the back of the eyeball by dissection, in fact, without even touching the eye!

Today's laser beams can be so accurately aimed and so sharply focused that with proper magnification they can cut a single cell in half — far finer than is needed for surgery on retinal tears. They are so powerful that they produce the desired effect in milliseconds (thousandths of a second). The apparatus is arranged to deliver the desired beam for the desired number of milliseconds automatically every time the surgeon aims and presses the trigger. Thus, like a sharpshooter using a telescopic gunsight to surround the bullseye, he can, in a few seconds, surround and seal a retinal tear with minute spot-welds and render it harmless. Since the bursts of light are of such short duration that they are barely seen or felt by the patient, this procedure can even be done with little or no anesthetic!

The above technique is more suitable for holes which are far enough back in the retina to be easily visible and accessible from the front (through the dilated pupil). Sometimes, tears near the front, at the edge of the retina, are not so easily seen or reached by the laser beam. For this, we now have another wonderful device.

Freezing

Some years ago animal research yielded the discovery that very low temperatures (30 to 70 degrees **below** zero centigrade) could produce adhering scars in tissues, somewhat like those produced by short-wave electric current or by light beams. Better still, it was soon found that such a freezing probe (cryoprobe) applied to the **outside** of the white of the eye could produce its "burn" and "scar" on the retina **inside** without burning the outside. So, by using the correct degree of freezing for the correct number of seconds, it is possible for the surgeon to surround some retinal tears with spot welds under local anesthesia without any cutting. Convalescence may take only a few days to a few weeks.

Meanwhile, back in the clinic and in the ophthalmologist's office, techniques for better diagnosis of smaller changes under greater magnification have been developed, so that it is now possible, with more high-powered ophthalmoscopes, to observe the finer structures of the retina with greater detail and precision than ever before. This leads us to an earlier and more accurate diagnosis and, when necessary, more meticulous and more successful surgery.

Summary

To summarize this chapter, let us return briefly to the patient with spots and flashes who comes, frightened, to the ophthalmologist's office. In nineteen patients out of twenty we find nothing of great importance and dismiss him or recheck him in a few days or weeks. We ask him meanwhile to avoid violent physical exertion or heavy lifting, so that if there is a weak spot, it is not traumatized and converted to a tear or a detachment.

In perhaps one patient out of twenty, we may discover an early retinal tear. If it is not yet detached, the retina around it can be spot-welded by means of light-coagulation, laser beam coagulation or freezing — under local anesthesia or no anesthesia, without hospitalization or at most a few days in hospital. There is a minimum of inconvenience and practically no discomfort. Best of all we have **prevented** a detachment and spared the patient a much more extensive and expensive operation, and, of course saved his sight.

If detachment has already occurred, surgery should be performed **without much** delay. With prompt operation, the outlook for successful reattachment is very good — about 95%. The prospect becomes poorer the longer the delay and the more extensive the detachment. In the great majority of reattached retinas, good vision is restored, except where the center of the retina (the macula) has been involved in the detachment, in which case only partial sight may be regained.

5
The Eyes of Children: The Crossed Eye and the Lazy Eye

They don't get better by themselves

Almost all "crossed eyes" (convergent strabismus) or "wall" eyes (divergent strabismus) can be straightened.

But —

Many of these eyes, though straightened, are left with defective vision (amblyopia).

Straightening the eyes is easy. Depending on circumstances, it can be done with glasses alone, or with drops, or with exercises, more often with combinations of these. If these methods are not effective, straightening by surgery is almost always successful. Operation can be performed at any age. However, a great many children whose eyes have been straightened, though improved in appearance, do not retain full sight of the two eyes. The child has a chance of keeping good sight only if treatment is started early. The later it is begun, the greater the likelihood that the child will be left with one poor eye. This is known as a "lazy" eye or, technically, amblyopia. We will discuss this first because it is the more important, then return to strabismus.

Amblyopia

The normal human uses the two eyes together because they point in the same direction. Both eyes focus on the same target at the same time. The brain perceives the two images coming from the two eyes as a single fused image. This is called binocular single vision.

When one eye is **out** of line, **its target** appears **displaced**. Therefore, the child sees **two** objects, one in **proper** position and one **displaced**. This is called double vision.

There are few sensations more disturbing than double vision. The infant with persistent double vision quickly cures his discomfort by ignoring the image of the crooked eye. We call this "suppression." In this way he no longer sees double because he has suppressed the disturbing second image. He is now comfortable because it is quite possible to get along using only one eye — a thousand times better than seeing double with two eyes. He literally teaches his brain not to perceive the second image by ignoring it, just as a few months earlier he taught it perception by seeing. Although he is now comfortable, the deviating eye does not develop good vision because it is not used.

I illustrate this in my office by showing the parents what it is like to have double vision (unless they, too, have one lazy eye — which is not uncommon because this condition tends to run in families). I ask them to look at any object, or at the vision chart, then I place a prism lens (wedge-shaped lens) before one eye. This artificially "crosses" the eye by slightly deflecting its line of sight, creating a second image. Invariably, the parent winces. Closing one eye restores comfortable single vision instantly. I then point out that the child does not go to the trouble of closing the eye but finds it easier to learn **not** to use it. But, I repeat, by doing so he fails to develop good vision in that eye.

The importance of early detection of amblyopia

The adult does not have the ability to 'suppress' one eye to eliminate double vision because during his entire life he has learned and firmly established a pattern of seeing well with **each** eye and with **both together**. Thus, if he suddenly develops strabismus, as sometimes happens when an eye muscle weakens from medical causes, he suffers greatly from double vision unless he closes one eye or covers it. If, instead, this had happened in infancy while the eye was still in the learning stage, he would not have needed to close one eye. Instead he would have, quite naturally, learned **not** to see — by ignoring it.

So we learn why early discovery of amblyopia is so important. The earlier discovered and corrected, the better and more firmly established will be the sight; the later, the more difficult will be any improvement. It is normal for the eyes to wander occasionally, up to the age of six months or even a year, because good muscle coordination may not yet have been well established. Any deviation **after** this time calls for an examination by an eye specialist.

No two children are alike. The specialist may, after examination, determine that for one child treatment should be deferred, while for another it must be started immediately. Such a decision involves many variable factors and should be made only by an expert. For the parent or even the pediatrician to decide whether to treat or wait is courting error. "Leave him alone, he'll grow out of it," often leaves one poor eye.

"Doctor, at what age should my child's eyes be examined?" is a question parents of apparently **normal** children ask. Ideally, at birth. The pediatrician includes the eyes as part of a complete medical examination of every child at birth and periodically thereafter. If he finds any abnormality he calls in the specialist.

Of course, certain tests cannot be performed, even by the specialist until the child is old enough to cooperate. This obviously differs in different children. Children under the age of twelve months cooperate too poorly for the more sophisticated tests. Where decisions of great importance depend on eye tests (such as with eye tumors or in infantile glaucoma) we may be compelled to examine the child under anesthesia. Fortunately, many amblyopias give us warning because the amblyopic eye is obviously out of line. But what about those children whose eyes are **not** obviously out of line?

The public has become more aware of amblyopia, thanks largely to the efforts of the National Society for the Prevention of Blindness. More and more screening is now done at pre-school age when detection is vitally important. What most parents do not know is that they need not be experts to test their own three or four year olds for amblyopia. In fact, such testing by a parent, done in a leisurely way and with patience, can be more valid than mass screening of large groups by a volunteer worker.

Home testing for amblyopia

A child need not know letters or numbers for his vision to be tested. Any parent can do this with any child of four or even three. All that is required is time and patience and above all a sense of "fun." Any inkling that this is a chore will result in resistance and inaccuracy. When well done, this test can be as accurate at home as in the ophthalmologist's office.

The test depends on the child learning to recognize the four positions of the letter **E** (**ɯ** , **m** , **ɘ** , **E**) and learning to show that he sees them by imitating their position, using his own two arms or the outstretched fingers of either hand. He learns this best by imitating a parent. The two parents, or one parent and an older sibling, play the "game" with one another in the **presence** of the infant but without (at first) allowing him to play. The exclusion is deliberate, on pretext of his being "too small." By being denied, he builds up an eagerness to play. This assures his attention and cooperation.

The **E** charts to be used should be cut (along the dotted line) from the five pages following page 68. The largest **E** is labelled on the back "for practice only." The successively smaller ones for testing are #1, #2, #3 and #4.

The parent stands ten feet from the child whose back is to a window or other source of light. Lighting should be adequate and need not be excessively bright. For the largest (practice) **E** neither eye should be covered at first, the motive being merely the learning of the four responses.

The parent shows the child the **E** turned in different directions. The child learns to respond by matching this direction with that of his own two arms or his fingers.

Take as much time as necessary. Do not exceed the normally short attention span. A few minutes daily is better than a long time once a week. If learning stretches over several weeks, don't worry — there is no hurry. Above all, let the occasion be fun rather than a chore. Never scold or criticize if wrong. Don't hesitate to help. Act pleasantly surprised if right; also praise and reward. With some children it is better to play the game only on special occasions or as a reward, thus associating it with something pleasant.

After he has learned to match the four directions, the process is repeated with one eye patched. He will not object if he has seen the parent wear a patch. Warning: If one eye is crossed, patch the **crossed** eye **first**. Patching the straight eye first may meet resistance if the crossed eye is amblyopic and not accustomed to seeing by itself.

An eye patch is better than the hand for covering one eye because the patch leaves both hands free. Opaque patches held in place by a string or rubber band can be bought or easily made at home out of cardboard. Make sure the child does not "peek" from behind the patch by twisting his head or tilting it so that he sees with the covered eye.

Note: When changing the position of the **E**, do not **rotate** it within sight of the child because this will enable him to rotate his hand in the same direction without seeing the **E**, but merely by watching the **direction** of the rotation. Instead, put the card down for an instant each time, then pick it up again, already turned in the new direction.

Vision of each eye is tested separately, beginning with the **E** chart #1, shown in different positions, then charts #2, 3 and 4. This is repeated for the other eye. On the accompanying blank form keep a written record of the smallest number **E** seen with each eye on a given date, as in the sample record below. You will need more charts, which you can easily make yourself.

Name			
Date	Smallest E Right Eye	Smallest E Left Eye	Remarks
Jan 5	# 1	# 4	Objects to covering left
Jan 11	# 2	# 4	Tries to peek, covers left
Jan 16	# 2	# 4	

Name			
Date	Smallest E Right Eye	Smallest E Left Eye	Remarks

Fig. 5. Sample Form and Blank Form for home testing for amblyopia.

If there is no consistent disparity between the two eyes, amblyopia is unlikely. If one eye is consistently poorer or if the child seems each time to object to covering the same eye or tries to peek, there may be amblyopia or some other condition which impairs the sight. Such a child should be examined by an eye specialist.

When you visit the specialist, bring with you the **E** charts you used and the record you kept. This will help him evaluate the child. Often the **E** tests done in the natural, relaxed home setting are more valid than those done in the doctor's office where the small child might be frightened and less cooperative.

Even if the eyes show no apparent abnormality, it is an easy and wise precaution for the parent to give this test to every child between the ages of three and four. There are instances of amblyopia **without** any crossing or other deviation. Children who are excessively far-sighted or very astigmatic may develop poor vision in one eye even though both eyes are straight. Other abnormalities, some of them curable, could be picked up earlier, if this test shows poor vision in one eye or a disparity between the two.

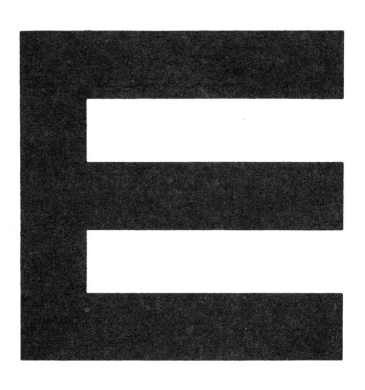

Ǝ

PRACTICE CHART

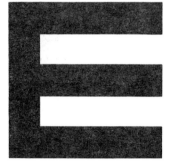

CHART 1

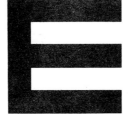

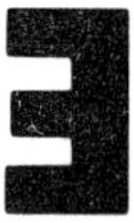

Ǝ

CHART 2

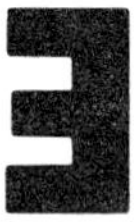

Ǝ

CHART 3

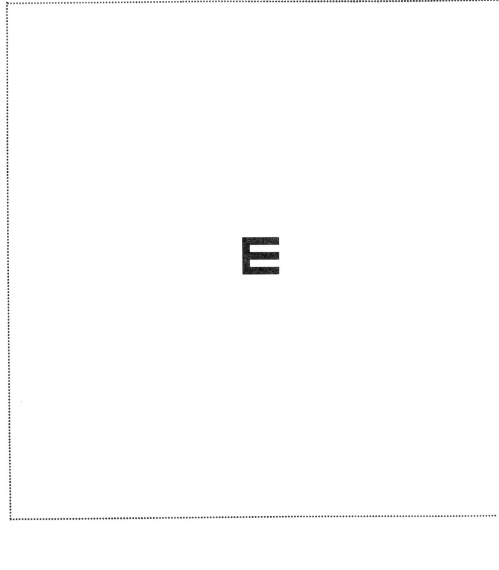

CUT ALONG DOTTED LINES

E

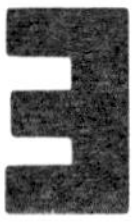

Ǝ

CHART 4

Strabismus

Strabismus is the general term applied to all abnormalities in coordination of the movements of the two eyes. The most common form is **convergent** strabismus (esotropia or esophoria) in which the eyes are "**crossed**" — deviated **inward**. Somewhat less common is **divergent** strabismus (exotropia or exophoria) — "**wall-eyed**" or deviated **outward**. Less common still but no rarity is an abnormal turn upward (hypertropia, hyperphoria). The distinction between "tropia" and "phoria" is that in the -tropia the eyes are deviated **constantly** and are never used together, while in the -phoria they deviate only **occasionally** and the rest of the time they are straight and work together. (Thus, in **esotropia** an eye is turned inward **all** of the time, in **esophoria** an eye is turned inward **occasionally**, and the rest of the time the eyes are straight and work together.)

Some children have "**alternating**" strabismus, meaning that **either** eye may turn, sometimes one, sometimes the other. Such children are less likely to have one amblyopic eye, but usually they still cannot use both eyes together.

Most strabismus becomes evident before the age of four years. Occasionally it is present very much earlier. Prior to one year of age, children's eyes may wander somewhat, possibly as a result of insufficiently developed muscle coordination rather than real strabismus; after one year or so, the normal eyes become straighter and remain so.

False strabismus

One frequent cause of false alarm is a condition known as **epicanthus**, which is present to a small degree in all infants. When it is more pronounced it makes the eyes **appear** crossed although in reality they are straight. Here is the explanation:

"Canthus" is the technical term for the corner or angle

where the upper and lower lids meet. Each eye has two corners: the lateral canthus (the outer corner) and the medial canthus (the inner corner). In the adult or in the older child, where the face has assumed more adult proportions, the inner and outer corners of each eye are about equally distant from the center of the pupil, so that the **same** amount of white is visible on **each** side of the eye. In the infant, the bridge of the nose appears wider and the inner corner is closer to the center of the pupil than is the outer corner (**epi**canthus = "above" the canthus). This causes less of the **white** of the eye to show on the side nearest the nose and creates the false impression that the eyes are crossed.

As the face grows, the bridge of the nose becomes narrower and the inner corner of each eye moves towards the bridge of the nose. Thus more of the white becomes visible on the nasal half of each eye and the child's eyes then appear straight. These are the children that "grow out" of the cross-eyedness because they were never really cross-eyed to begin with. They are the source of the legend that cross-eyed children "grow out of it." The real ones usually don't. If you have any doubt whether your child's strabismus is false or real, he should be examined by an eye specialist.

Crossed eyes occur more commonly in far-sighted children; divergent eyes in near-sighted ones. Both types are more common in families where the condition has existed in ancestors or siblings. For this reason, children in such families should be examined by an ophthalmologist early in life to rule out amblyopia even if strabismus is not obvious. And, after age three or four, the Home Test for amblyopia should be attempted.

The treatment of strabismus

The treatment of strabismus is almost always successful

if begun at the proper time, if the parents are cooperative and if the child is not too resistant to patching or glasses when necessary.

It is impossible to outline details of treatment for each case. As I have said, this book is not a substitute for the doctor. No book can possibly anticipate and meet every variation which can occur in every individual case. There are as many variations as there are children and only the expert, after careful examination, can tell what to do for a particular child.

The following will merely help you cooperate more intelligently with your doctor by laying down certain principles. It will also give you a number of hints on how to follow your doctor's instructions in order to make your task at home easier and more effective.

The treatment of strabismus has four objectives:

1. Prevention of amblyopia
2. Straightening of the eyes
3. Preventing the devastating psychological effect on the child's personality of such facial deformity
4. Where possible, making the eyes work together.

Amblyopia has already been discussed, as has been the importance of early detection. Its treatment usually consists of forcing the lazy eye into use, either by straightening the deviated eye so that it naturally begins to work together with the straight eye, or by interfering with the straight eye so that the child is compelled to employ the lazy eye. Your doctor will decide which to do first, depending on what is best and most feasible in the individual case.

If he decides that interfering with the good eye should come first, it is usually done by blocking devices which range all the way from special lenses which cut out only part of the sight to total occluders which block all use of the good eye. These can be of various materials, applied in different ways and worn either constantly or intermittently, depending on the doctor's instructions.

Some very small children readily accept blocking the good eye; others resist violently. Tact, diplomacy and patience will usually prevail; occasionally the parent must resort to force. In general, the younger the child the less likely he is to resist patching. Conversely, the older the child and the longer the vision of the poor eye has been suppressed, the more strongly he resists blocking the good eye.

A very young child may more readily accept an eye patch if he sees the parent or others in the family wearing one. Another trick is to first patch the child's **defective** eye — the eye which he does not use and will not miss. This accustoms him to the idea of **any** patch at all, without impairing his ability to see, then to switch the patch to the good eye.

Again, the more he resists, the more it is an indication of how poor the eye is, and how badly it needs to be stimulated by patching the good one.

In rare instances, the child will not yield to reason, persuasion or bribery, and repeatedly tears off the occluder. Here restraint may be necessary in the form of splinting both elbows, using light strips of wood, plastic or cardboard. The simplest splint is made from a thin piece of cardboard, about 8 by 16 inches in size, wound twice around the child's arm from 4 inches above the elbow to 4 inches below the elbow, then fastened in place by taping it to the sleeve. This allows the child free movement of the arms, wrists, hands and fingers but prevents him from bending his elbow to bring his hand to his face and tearing off the eye patch. Admittedly an extreme measure, it is used mostly on very small children only when there is extreme resistance. It usually needs to be continued for only a short time until the child learns that tearing off the patch only brings another period of splinting.

Rarely, there are children whose amblyopia is so profound and whose resistance is so stubborn that nothing seems to help. In such instances, or where there are other physical or emotional reasons for not pursuing the matter further, the parent must accept the fact that the child will grow up with one amblyopic eye. Although this is unfortunate, it is not the castastrophe it would seem to be because it is quite possible to live a normal life with only one perfect eye. Millions of people have done so (see Chapter 10).

Mothers often want to know how safe it is for the child to get about with only the amblyopic eye when the good eye is covered. The answer to this will vary greatly with the individual child and with the extent and previous duration of the amblyopia. The older child may have much difficulty for the first few days or even weeks, especially if he had been allowed to reach school age before the amblyopia was discovered.Such a child may need watching or some help at first. In most cases the difficulty is not too great because amblyopia usually impairs only the sharper central vision for fine detail but leaves peripheral vision unimpaired. Thus, such a child would probably see well enough to walk about, to detect approaching people, bicycles or cars but (at first) be unable to read, discern license plates or faces. I instruct the parent to watch over him when the good eye is first patched to see how well he performs at home before going outdoors unaccompanied and before wearing a patch at school. Improvement is often rapid.

It is important that the parent clearly understand which eye is the one to be patched. Occasionally the mother misunderstands and the amblyopic eye is patched by mistake. This does no harm except for the nuisance and the loss of a few weeks' time. It can be avoided by making sure at the time of the visit to the ophthalmologist's office which eye to patch.

Sometimes a mother telephones, much concerned because she has patched the good eye for a few weeks and she now notices that on removing the patch for bedtime it is the **good** eye which is **crossed** and the poor eye which is straight. This, I assure her, is an excellent sign that the occlusion has been successful and the child's amblyopic eye so much improved that he sees sufficiently well to want to use it. Patching has cured only the amblyopia but the strabismus remains. Since one eye still has to cross, seeing with the crossed eye will, at the moment, naturally force the **good** eye to **cross**. In other words, the strabismus which formerly affected only one eye has now been improved to an **alternating** strabismus — the child can see with either eye. The next step is to make the eyes straight.

The actual straightening of the eyes may be accomplished in a number of ways. The methods used and the sequence, timing and age will be determined by the eye specialist, based on what is best in each individual instance. In the great majority, success may be predicted with confidence.

Glasses

Some children with strabismus can be cured merely by wearing glasses. This is especially true of far sighted ones with convergent strabismus and of near-sighted ones with divergent strabismus. Usually the eye specialist will use "drops" to measure more accurately the extent of the need for glasses. He will also take advantage of the dilated pupils to examine the interior of the eyes more carefully. In this way he makes certain that there is not some other cause for poor vision and for the strabismus.

Exercises

Exercises, alone or combined with glasses, are often recommended for straightening the eyes in certain types of strabismus. There are many kinds of exercises, tailored to meet different needs. The entire field of eye muscle and vision training, known as orthoptics, has become an important branch of ophthalmology and optometry. Many ophthalmologists and optometrists do their own orthoptic work when a child requires it. Some practitioners or clinics use orthoptists, people especially trained to do orthoptics — to work with them in teaching the children to improve coordination of eye movements.

Various kinds of apparatus are employed in this effort. Some are so simple that the parent and child can be taught to use them at home; others are too elaborate to be used outside the office and must be controlled by the ophthalmologist himself or by an orthoptist.

Orthoptic exercises may also be used before and/or after surgery to enhance the cooperation of the two eyes.

Drops

Certain types of strabismus respond favorably to drops, either alone or in conjunction with glasses or exercises. Whether to use them, and when, will be determined by the ophthalmologist.

Surgery

Surgery is often the easiest, quickest and surest way to straighten the child's eyes, and it is, in some instances, quite proper to do this at the outset. In most cases, however, glasses and/or exercises or drops are tried first; if not successful, surgery is then performed.

The principle of this surgery is quite simple: the

correction of the muscle imbalance which has been keeping the eyes out of line. The proper muscles are reset or shortened or lengthened with sufficient precision to straighten the eyes. Operation may be on one or both eyes; anywhere from one to four muscles may be adjusted at one stage. In some cases, only partial correction (undercorrection) is sought, with more to be done later if necessary.

While most other eye operations involve the interior of the eyeball, all surgery on the **eye muscles** is performed **outside** the eyeball because that is where the muscles are — within the socket, but outside the globe. Thus, although they are delicate and precise, eye muscle operations are among the easiest and safest performed by eye surgeons. Complications are slight and very rare.

Because almost all the patients are children and certain to be frightened, surgery is performed under general anesthesia. In adults, local anesthesia is quite adequate. In either case, there is no pain.

In all cases, convalescence is rapid, discomfort is minimal (although the eye may remain red for a number of weeks) and the results are usually excellent.

Results

In summary, I can only reiterate that almost all strabismus cases can be cured. This is gratifying not only to the child and the parents but to the eye surgeon as well.

The blessings achieved are threefold:

If amblyopia is prevented or cured, the child ends up with two functioning eyes instead of only one. In the rare instances of eye injury this could give him a second eye to fall back on.

If the eyes are straight enough to achieve binocular vision and depth perception, he has better use of them than would be the case with only monocular vision. In the modern world, with its demand for highly skilled performance, these attributes can make the difference between success and failure.

Third, and perhaps most rewarding of all, is the effect on the child's personality. It is an almost daily source of delight to see children who used to cringe and withdraw because of their deformed appearance and the taunts of their playmates, become outgoing and cheerful as soon as their eyes have been straightened.

It is exciting enough to restore the sight of an aging person for his remaining years by removing his cataracts. How much more of a thrill it is to restore the morale of a child whose whole life lies before him!

6
The Eyes of Children: Other Common Problems

The red eye

Most of what you will want to know about inflamed eyes in children can be found in Chapter 9 on the inflamed eye. That chapter applies to children as well as to adults.

But children differ from adults in a number of ways which necessitate greater vigilance on the part of parents and greater ingenuity by the doctor.

Small children often do not complain of what is disturbing them. They haven't the experience to know what is abnormal. Granted, if there is severe pain, they cry and may even rub the eyes, but crying is often ascribed to colic or teething, while rubbing can be a natural part of crying. Most eye conditions are more subtle and do not evoke crying. The very young infant with cataract, glaucoma or an obstructed tear duct does not know that diminished vision or tearing is wrong.

The younger the child, the less able he is to describe his distress in words. It is only after the child is old enough to talk that he can say "Mommy, my eye hurts," or "the light hurts," and very much older before he is likely to recognize blurring of vision — and, at that, only if it is **sudden** and involves **both** eyes. **Gradual** blurring, especially if it affects **only one** eye, often goes unrecognized, even in adults.

Therefore, because children do not often sound the alarm, parents must be all the more alert to any signs of eye trouble. They can do this only if they know what they are:

Some signs of eye trouble

Redness of one or both eyes, especially if persistent and not due to crying or to an obvious cold.

Tearing, constant or intermittent of one or both eyes, not due to crying or an obvious cold. Be careful here: it may not be a cold; tearing from inflamed eyes could mimic a cold because tears flowing down into the nose through the tear ducts could keep the nose running. (See also the section on obstruction of tear ducts in infants, further on in this chapter.)

Discharge of pus or mucus from one or both eyes, with or without pasting or crusting of the eyelids.

Sensitivity to light: the infant winces or squeezes the lids shut or tries to avoid light or bury his face.

Obvious inability to see as in failure to follow a light or a moving object or, later, recognize a parent by sight and not by voice or footstep.

Frequent scowling, squinting, rubbing of the eyes could mean disease.

Obvious strabismus or head-tilt (see Chapter 5 on strabismus; also false strabismus).

Pronounced disparity in the size of the two pupils. Minute differences are usually of little consequence (but call them to the attention of your pediatrician during your next visit to him). Large pupils are normal for most children but they should contract moderately in bright flashlight or sunlight. However, noticeable difference in size of the two pupils may mean trouble.

Any whitish or yellowish reflection from behind either pupil should be investigated. It may have no significance or it may mean cataract or tumor. Such conditions are not common in infants but they can occur.

Any one or combination of the above symptoms, especially if they are accompanied by evidence of discomfort, should be seen by the pediatrician or by the eye specialist.

The examination and treatment of children's eyes

The examination and treatment of children calls for much greater ingenuity on the part of the doctor, to say nothing of tact, gentleness and patience.

We have already seen that the younger the child, the less able he is to describe his symptoms. There is, of course, none of the cooperation we take for granted in adults, and tests requiring such cooperation simply cannot be done. In addition, he is frightened by the new surroundings and the lights. Mercifully, this is less so in infants under the age of four or five months who are still not smart enough to be frightened.

This can be turned into an advantage. Contrary to what most parents think, some examinations and treatments are **easier** when infants are so very young. They are not aware of what is going on and they can be diverted by the only important event in their lives — feeding. Accordingly I ask parents to bring the child at feeding time and withhold the bottle until he is good and hungry. If drops must be used either for local anesthesia or for dilating the pupils, they can be instilled before the examination or even at home before leaving for the office. I have resorted to this method countless times, even for such procedures as irrigating an obstructed tear duct to cure persistent tearing. Examination for such extremely rare conditions as infantile cataract, retinal tumor, or infantile glaucoma often can also be carried out in the same way.

After five months of age, my "milk bottle anesthesia" becomes progressively less effective, and most children are at their most resistant between eighteen months and two years. At that age a mild sedative (after checking with the pediatrician) is sometimes helpful, and in extreme cases where a thorough examination is imperative, one must consider a light, brief general anesthesia.

Tearing in new born infants

A brief word about tearing in very small infants because it is so common and because most cases can be cured easily if treated early:

Some babies are born with obstruction of one or both tear ducts. (For a description of tear ducts, see p. 217.) The ducts may be narrower than normal, or, more usually, contain mucous plugs which block the proper flow of tears out of the eye and down into the nose. Because of the absence of a passageway, there may also be an accumulation of pus in the eye and a tendency for the lids to become pasted together during sleep. Some of the pus, mucus and tear fluid may even collect in the tear sac causing it to swell and form a small lump just below the nasal corner of the eyelids.

In a few instances, the obstructions clear spontaneously and the tearing stops. In hope of this, it is safe to wait a few weeks (if the tear sac is not badly swollen). Unfortunately, some parents wait many months, thinking that treatment will be easier if the infant is older. The opposite is true — it is easier before the age of four months. The eye specialist may then reestablish a passageway by massaging the tear sac or by gently flushing the duct through a tiny tube inserted while the child is taking his bottle — a procedure which is painless and may not even interrupt his feeding, except perhaps to startle him and make him gulp when some of the salt solution floods into his nose and mouth and mixes with the milk he swallows.

If the parents delay until the child is older, the "milk bottle anesthesia" is not as effective. Restraint or even anesthesia is then necessary. In the rare instance that the obstruction is more profound and does not yield to irrigation, it may be necessary to widen the tear duct by means of a minor operation under general anesthesia.

Eye injuries in children

Every parent should read the chapter on eye injuries and the prevention of blindness, which applies to children as well as adults. Statistically, the chances are your child will never sustain an eye injury. But if he should, it will be better to have read that chapter beforehand. It may even **prevent** an accident.

Children who hold books too close

Sometimes children between third and seventh grades are brought to my office because they read with the printed page held too close to their eyes.

A few have some abnormality or need glasses. But the majority turn out, after careful examination, to have no eye disease and to be neither near-sighted nor astigmatic.

The problem is mostly psychological, based either on lack of confidence because reading is still a relatively new experience, or on the habit acquired in the first grade of being accustomed to reading large-type print. In the higher grades, text book print is smaller. But the child feels more comfortable with the type as large as formerly. He makes it larger by holding it closer.

When I am satisfied the child's vision is normal, I show the parent how adequately the child reads ordinary type at arm's length. This convinces both of them that no glasses are necessary.

Almost all these children, if left alone, read at normal distance after they have acquired more skill and confidence. If given glasses unnecessarily, they soon start forgetting to wear them. They are right — they did not need them in the first place.

Incidentally, this is why some people falsely assume that children can be cured of near-sightedness early by wearing glasses for a few months. These children were not near-sighted and there was nothing to cure.

Eyestrain in children: the importance of physical activity

Some children suffer from eyestrain because of prolonged and incessant studying, reading or television unrelieved by any physical activity. The younger the child, the more physical activity he requires. Were it not for school, children in the natural state, like young animals, would be almost constantly on the move. We quite properly put them in school six hours a day, but the afternoons should be set aside for free play with vigorous use of the larger muscles. Homework and television are better left for the evening.

I have noticed much more eyestrain among children in the last twenty-five years and it is usually in those children who do not play outdoors after school but do homework or watch television, then do more of the same in the evening.

How much television should children watch?

It is almost impossible to generalize because children vary so much. Other factors also vary, such as the presence of other eye problems, the quality of the image on the TV set, and how well rested the child is.

Usually, when asked, I recommend not more than one hour a day if the child watches every day, two to three hours if viewing is limited to week-ends.

In my own experience, a very approximate rule of thumb is that one hour of television causes an amount of eye fatigue equivalent to two or two and a half hours of movies, i.e., in a regular motion-picture theater. Movies are more painstakingly put together with more attention to photography, sharpness of image, better contrasts, less abrupt changes of scene, etc., and a larger, brighter and better focused image, permitting the child to sit much further away from the screen than from the TV set.

In fact, distance between child and set is as important as duration of viewing. A child should sit at least six feet away, preferably eight. Aside from being less strain at greater distance, there is the small possibility of stray short-wave radiation from some sets, especially color TV, at distances closer than six feet. Whether or not such exposure is harmful has not yet been clearly established. Until we know more definitely, I therefore recommend keeping the child at least six feet away.

During television viewing, it is best to avoid total darkness. Even a small light in another part of the room is enough.

Near-sightedness in children

Near-sighted children often become more near-sighted during the years of their most rapid growth. It is not unusual for them to require stronger glasses as often as every six months, outgrowing the glasses with every inch they gain in height.

This is often a source of concern to parents who reason that the process will go on indefinitely, but I assure them that it is in some way connected with growth and will probably level off when the child has reached full height.

Heredity is also an influencing factor. Myopia is often inherited and if both parents are myopic the tendency to increasing myopia is greater.

Years ago myopic children were encouraged to avoid reading and in extreme cases they were actually kept out of school. Today the prevailing opinion is that ordinary reading or school work, even in large amounts, makes little difference. Also, whether or not glasses are worn does not affect the rate of change.

Most near-sighted people live normal lives and their only handicap is the nuisance of being dependent on glasses or contact lenses. The nuisance may become an advantage when they are able to read without glasses at middle age and beyond, a time when their normal or far-sighted contemporaries find it necessary to put on glasses for reading. Near-sightedness is usually the secret behind the aged grandparent who "can still read or thread a needle without glasses."

7
The Eyes of Children: Why Johnny Can't Read

Learning to read is not often a medical or ophthalmo-logical problem, but is usually the concern of the educator and the psychologist. What is it doing in a book like this? The fact is that over the years a great many children have been brought to me in the hope that correction of an ocular problem will make them good readers.

Intrigued by the challenge, I studied the subject in some depth from the point of view of the ophthalmologist. I also learned a great deal from my little patients and their parents. In some instances I was actually able to help. Even in failure I found the problem fascinating despite (or because) so little is really known and so much of what is accepted is contra-dictory or unproven.

Of course most children **can** read, and do read very well. But this is small consolation to the parents of those children who have a frustrating inability to read, an inability often **un**related to vision, to other aptitudes or to general intelligence. The condition is known by a number of confusing names. You may have heard of dyslexia, faulty perception and other terms.

The prevalence of reading disability
There is even confusion over what constitutes reading disability and how much of it exists. Researchers have

published varying statistics, based on different criteria, that between 5% and 35% of all school children have reading difficulties. One need not be a sociologist to understand the impact of such widespread disability on a highly technical society like ours. It influences employability, mental health, intelligent voting, poverty, crime — not to mention the staggering cost of vainly trying to impart a conventional academic education in a conventional manner to so many children who cannot read or who cannot make sense out of what they do read.

What is the effect of reading disability on the individual child? The best single word to describe it is "frustration." Aside from the educational and occupational handicaps — which are bad enough — the emotional trauma resulting from inadequacy and failure can be devastating, especially in modern times when the emphasis is on education for advanced technology, and when the jobs which used to provide fulfillment for the less skilled are now being performed by machines.

In today's egalitarian society, children are under pressure from various sources to attend high school and college. In the rural setting of former years, it was socially acceptable and easy for those not academically oriented to leave school and become artisans, laborers, mechanics, merchants or even executives. They thus found satisfaction and economic security in their own place in society. Today, instead of productive and reasonably secure manual workers or tradesmen, we have an increasing number of young people whose attempts to cope with formal education lead only to frustration, with all its emotional and sociological side-effects, and who end up as drop-outs anyway.

Causes of reading disability

Some reading problems are due to genuine dyslexia — a defect which, in the current state of our knowledge, must be considered extremely difficult, and sometimes impossible to correct. We will discuss it presently but first let us touch on a few other causes which might hold out some hope of relief and some which might even be preventable. What are these other causes?

Medical

    Poor vision

    Poor hearing

    Other medical problems

Psychological

    Reading block

    Other psychological problems

    Cultural deprivation

    Lack of motivation

    Television

Dyslexia

Obviously, in many children several of these causes may be present or overlapping and interacting.

Poor vision

Nowadays, if the child has poor vision, it is usually discovered before he enters first grade. The family doctor and the pediatrician look for abnormalities in the infant's eyes at birth or shortly afterward. If any are found, he is referred to the eye specialist. Again before entering school or kindergarten, most communities require an eye test, or better still, an eye examination.

However, there is a three year period, between the ages of two and five, when important abnormalities might be overlooked. This is both unnecessary and a great pity because during this critical period such defects can be detected at home by the parents long before their children are able to recognize numbers or letters. I refer to two conditions known as amblyopia or "lazy" eye, and strabismus, or "crossed" eye. They are discussed in detail in Chapter 6. In that chapter the parents will also find charts and instructions for their use at home in detecting amblyopia. Either condition, as soon as discovered, should be placed under the care of an eye specialist for early treatment and cure.

However, when it comes to reading problems, poor vision, even amblyopia or strabismus, are themselves rarely the cause of difficulty in reading. A child may do poorly in school if his near-sightedness or astigmatism is uncorrected and he cannot see the blackboard; or if he is cross-eyed and the taunts of his classmates make him withdrawn. But none of these is usually the immediate cause of poor reading — much to the disappointment of parents who had hoped that glasses or exercises or surgery to straighten the eyes would solve the reading problem too. I have seen a great many children with less than acceptable vision, or with one amblyopic eye, who were nevertheless good readers and who went on to do well in advanced education. In fact, it used to be that those whose poor vision prevented them from participating in outdoor games were the "bookworms." In the days before television, they often became the scholars, writers, and researchers despite their need to work harder in the seeing process.

A warning about eye exercises

A word about eye exercises to improve poor reading: It is a simple matter for the ophthalmologist to determine whether the child has any eye muscle abnormalities or imbalances and whether these will be helped by exercises. If so, they can be very effective. Sometimes there is doubt and he may suggest trying them. Usually they do not help if the eye muscles are not the cause of the reading difficulty. I have known many parents who persisted in subjecting their children to eye exercises, as a last resort or because they wanted something concrete attempted. Where the ophthalmologist has found no need for "eye exercises," they almost invariably, after many months of scolding and expense, turn out to be a waste of time and effort.

Defective hearing

Similarly, defective hearing should be ruled out by the pediatrician. If in doubt, an otologist (ear specialist) should be consulted. Correction of faulty hearing can markedly improve a child's classroom work. It is even more important long before school age, because much of the child's language skill on which reading and learning are based depends on good hearing early in life.

Other medical problems

Medical conditions are sometimes the cause of difficulty in reading or learning. Fortunately, many of them can be easily discovered by the pediatrician or family doctor. They include mild diabetes, malnutrition, anemia, intestinal parasites, thyroid disturbance, the taking of drugs. The family physician or pediatrician may also want to enlist the aid of a neurologist in discovering mild epileptic seizures which may not be sufficiently pronounced for parents or teachers to notice, yet are discernible on neurological examination and encephalogram. Many of the above respond to appropriate treatment, often with gratifying improvement in reading and learning. The neurologist will also look for evidence of cerebral insufficiency, sometimes called minimum brain damage. None of the above tests causes the least pain or discomfort.

Reading block

I have examined many children over the years whose poor reading has turned out to be the result of block — psychological block, also known as reading inhibition — caused by too much pressure from parent or teacher, applied too early or too crudely in an effort to make them read as well as their peers. These little ones are often bright, verbal, interested and outgoing although some become sullen and defensive. The natural history of reading block often runs as follows:

A child may read a bit more slowly than his classmates. Some first-grade children, especially boys, catch on later than others. This is referred to technically as maturational lag. An overzealous teacher may single out this child as a "poor reader" and his troubles begin. The teacher, the parent, the psychologist, the special reading teacher — all zero-in on him. The frightened child soon becomes convinced of his inadequacy. He learns only to dread reading. It is possible that if such a child had been left alone he might have been reading as well as his peers by the end of the year.

I have seen six year olds who were barely in the first grade and who, with no evidence of dyslexia, had already been labelled poor readers. It always reminds me of the child who was disgraced by the report of a fussy kindergarten teacher because he was "deficient in pasting"!

Dealing with reading block

The small child singled out as a poor reader may remain

a poor reader unless help is given in a casual and relaxed atmosphere. Psychological block, once established, is difficult to overcome. The only hope of breaking this cycle of pressure—resistance—more pressure—more resistance, is to stop the pressure. If it comes from the parent, he should "lay off." This is not always easy because he wants his child to excel. It helps if he understands that the gung-ho spirit that works on the little league baseball team may be just wrong for tackling first grade reading. Where pressure comes from a well-meaning but over-zealous teacher, a good deal depends on her flexibility and understanding once the problem has been explained. Most teachers are cooperative, but it is occasionally necessary to make a complete change to a different class, and in extreme cases, to a new school or even a new neighborhood.

On the other hand, human beings don't always follow the rules. Results sometimes surprise us. I recall vividly how, years ago, I scolded a colleague of mine because he was literally locking his small son in his room until all homework was done! I warned of dire consequences. Today, that son is — guess what — a famous neurosurgeon. But that father was just lucky; his method was just the right one for producing a drop-out. Had the boy been more sensitive, more individualistic, more independent (and these can be powerful traits if nurtured gently) he might have resisted the pressure by developing a block against reading and studying.

Other psychological problems

The presence of other emotional or psychiatric disturbances sufficient to interfere with reading and learning should be evaluated by the psychologist or psychiatrist in cooperation with the parents, the pediatrician, or the family doctor. The teacher or the social worker might in some instances be able to provide more information relative to the child's background, environment and home stresses than the parents. It is, of course, possible that personality deviations could be the result rather than the cause of reading difficulty. In some cases, counselling and/or therapy could bring about improvement. But this, like medical problems, should be in the hands of experts.

Cultural deprivation

Don't skip this topic because you are not poor. You don't have to be "disadvantaged" to "enjoy" cultural deprivation — and for your child to start life similarly deprived.

Children respond to the people around them. They are the world's greatest imitators. It is almost funny to see small children unconsciously reproduce a parent's mannerisms, speech, gait or posture. So if you want your child to be a good reader — and with few exceptions this is the key to being a good student — you must do something about it. This starts not with first grade or kindergarten or even nursery school. It starts with you in the home, in the nursery.

Second only to love and a feeling of security and belonging, an infant's intellectual development requires communication, and this almost from birth! The fact that he cannot talk and answer and that he sleeps sixteen hours a day does not mean that when awake he is not receiving and absorbing impressions — and language. Some day we will be able to prove that children learn at a greater rate **before** age one or two than afterward.

So, talk to him. Right from the beginning, in addition to loving him, talk to him. Not surprisingly, the one fact that I remember from reading Thomas Wolfe's "Look Homeward Angel" forty years ago was his description of how incessantly his father spoke to the children whenever he was at home. Wolfe's books show it!

The infant who is asleep by the time the commuting father comes home, and whose mother is too busy working or participating in community affairs, the infant who is regarded as a burden to be turned over to a stranger merely to be kept fed, dry, tidy and out of mischief but rarely spoken to except in admonition (the story of the child who said his name was "Hey, You" is sadder than it is funny) — such an infant is being more intellectually deprived than if he were kept out of first grade until age nine!

I think that much of a feel for language may be acquired long before the child is able to speak. Perhaps being only an ophthalmologist and not a psychologist, I have no right to propose such a theory. But I base it on something I do know: the cause of amblyopia — the failure to develop good vision from lack of use **in early childhood**. (See Chapter 5 on amblyopia.) Could one not postulate that a language sense may fail to develop in the same way? In fact, some authorities consider it possible that true dyslexia may come from non-stimulation at a critical stage, resulting in the failure to develop certain communication centers in the brain. Could this be some form of cerebral amblyopia? And preventable?

So, you have been talking to him. What is the next obvious step? Of course: Read to him! He need not understand every word. Next to cuddling and play, the small child loves to be read to. Don't be afraid to comply when he pleads, "Read it again." He's merely asking for an encore because he enjoyed it. Don't be surprised if he fills in what you omit. When the child is three, or four, or five he will often "read" the same stories himself, or even out loud, to you. Pretend that he is really reading rather than reciting from memory. Then one day soon, he **will** really be reading if enough simple stuff is left around and he is not prodded to read. Unless there is something else very much wrong, such a child will have no trouble in the first grade — except perhaps boredom. And if he has been in the habit of seeing one or both parents habitually sitting and reading for their own pleasure, he may also continue the practice and grow up to be a reader.

Lack of motivation

A normal child reacts to an incessant stream of stimuli via all his senses during all his waking hours. Unless blocked, he is curious about everything. One might say that he is instinctively motivated to learn. As any parent knows, he is virtually tireless. Given love, security, nourishment and shelter, the process of learning goes on endlessly, feeding on itself and branching out almost without limit. He soon discovers that reading is another means of further satisfying this curiosity.

A child's motivation, like his intellectual development, is best stimulated in the home. More time and attention spent with the child in the early years by interested — and interesting — parents who are not too busy to answer questions and to offer intellectual challenges judiciously and lightly, without overpowering his mental capacity, his short attention span or his sense of freedom to explore in his own way, — all can help establish a pattern of eager and open-eyed response to the world around him and motivate him to continue learning once he is in school.

Television

Television impedes not only reading, but speech as well. The small child learns to speak by speaking. This is a prelude to learning to read by reading. The television offers the opportunity only to listen but not to talk back. Children become passive spectators rather than active participants.

When I went to grade school, before the invention of radio and TV, evenings and rainy days were spent reading; there was nothing else to do. The line for the children's room at the public library extended far out into the street. Today, too many children find it easier to be entertained by TV at the flick of a switch than to work at reading. It has been my experience over the last twenty-five years (since television) that a much higher proportion of my young patients now read less fluently and speak badly. It is no wonder: a recent survey showed that many seventeen year olds have spent more time watching TV than attending school. In fact they have spent more time in front of the tube than in any other single activity except sleep.

On the other hand, television has enormous potential for providing the proper stimulation of school children by presenting interesting and subtle programs designed more for education than for selling cereals. Even where such programs exist — and they are all too few — they are obliged to compete for the school audience with others that are pure junk but are more lurid and exciting. If the public could see its way to providing a mere few million for truly educational, non-commercial TV, it could save hundreds of times as much money now being spent on remedial measures for older children whose creativity and ingenuity had been stifled by trash at a crucial period in their early development.

Dyslexia

What do we mean by dyslexia?

The interesting fact is that no one is really quite sure. The large number of other names for it is a measure of the confusion: poor reading, faulty perception, reading disability, learning disability, retarded reader, retarded learner, congenital word blindness, developmental dyslexia, primary developmental dyslexia, strephosymbolia. These terms are not synonymous, but for simplicity we will group them together. The scientific papers and books that have been written about them over the past eighty years by educators, psychologists, psychiatrists, sociologists, neurologists and ophthalmologists would fill a small library. Their definitions and the differences among them are often obscure; theories regarding causes and cures are contradictory. The voluminous literature and the many conflicting theories themselves indicate how little is firmly known on the subject. Much of what is generally accepted is still unproven.

What the parent wants is not theory, but a description of the condition and what, if anything, he can do about it. He is already aware that his child's problem will not be solved by the novice and is quite willing to leave the technical details to the expert. So I hope I am forgiven if I oversimplify.

In this discussion I shall use the term "dyslexia" which is Latin for "difficulty with words." This is appropriate precisely because it is less specific and especially because, if one must use any term in the presence of a small child, this one is less crushing than "learning disability," or "retarded learner," or "poor reader." And who can pronounce "strephosymbolia?"

What are the signs of dyslexia?

Children with dyslexia may vary greatly but they have one thing in common: poor reading — often despite other attributes, such as good intelligence, background and motivation, which should make them **good** readers. (The generally retarded, and severely disturbed children whose other problems overshadow their reading difficulties cannot be included in this discussion.) Children with dyslexia may have difficulty in perceiving what others see or hear; or in distinguishing one letter or word from another. Some cannot recognize letters or words well enough to remember them, organize them or make sense of them. Some cannot learn to read by the "sight method." Their reading is laborious, they cannot remember whole-word patterns, they are poor spellers and poor oral readers. In the early learning stages, there may be confused orientation of letters (b-d; p-q) and words (saw-was, felt-left, on-no) and numbers (12-21). This is sometimes referred to as "mirror-reading." (Still, I have seen children with similar confused orientation in the early stages of learning who were not true dyslexics and who by the time they had reached third grade, became good readers.)

On tests of perception which employ drawing or copying of geometric patterns, their figures tend to be more primitive and fluid — squares become rounded, oblique lines become vertical or horizontal and vice versa; open figures may be closed. Children with dyslexia may also (but not necessarily) display poor motor coordination — as in handwriting, dexterity or sports. Yet there are dyslexics who draw well and poor draughtsmen who are very good readers. And experts do not agree on the relationship between dyslexia and left-handedness or poor one-sided motor preference.

There may be other language problems such as delayed

or imperfect speech, poor oral vocabulary, or a bad ear for words. Some do poorly in arithmetic but others do well and even go on to excel in mathematics.

They may have emotional problems and sometimes it is not clear whether these are part of the picture of dyslexia or the result of the frustration therefrom. The attention span is short; they are easily distracted and unable to concentrate on any subject for long; they are overactive, flitting from one task to another and may act or speak impulsively without regard to consequences. Emotionally unstable, they bear criticism or failure badly and often feel rejected by their peers, their teachers and their parents although they seem to seek attention and acceptance. However, many dyslexics are emotionally stable.

You begin to see how much uncertainty and contradiction surround the subject. There is more. There are various degrees of dyslexia. Some are so slight that the diagnosis is obscure. In the most severe cases, the child finds it impossible to distinguish one letter or word from another.

What causes dyslexia?

Why does dyslexia afflict certain children who seem otherwise normal? No one really knows. Some theories hold that it is the failure in development of certain pathways, connections or centers in the brain concerned with the intricate process of sight, recognition, and interpretation. No one knows whether this occurs before birth, while the brain structures of the embryo are still taking shape — something like what happens in German measles at certain stages of pregnancy — or after birth when the pathways already formed are not put to use at the precise time they should be "learning" to work. Much research still needs to be done on this and related subjects before we even begin to understand, prevent or cure. We do know that dyslexia is more than three times as common in males than in females and that in some families the condition tends to show up in successive generations.

Reading, and its more advanced purpose, learning, involve much more than "seeing." The simple act of seeing — viewing an object by the normal eye so that its image is accurately focused on the retina, ready for transmission to the brain — this act in itself is one of the wonders of nature. Yet, it is primitive compared to the entire learning process. The sharp sight of the hawk is legendary, but the hawk cannot read.

The conversion of this basic first step into learning is ever so much more sophisticated. It requires the need to recognize letters and words once they have been seen, to remember them, to orient them, group them, organize them in meaningful sequences. And in the more advanced processes — to interpret, to form concepts, to deduce, to theorize and to reason abstractly.

Even the mere physical transmission of the visual stimulus required in the reading process is enormously intricate. From the retina the image is flashed by way of a complicated pathway of nerve fibers through several relays to the visual center at the very back of the brain, called the occiput. The occiput has many sensory areas. These areas have been mapped out and numbered. It is in area number 17, a reception center, that the image first appears. From here it is sent by another set of microscopic nerve connections to areas 18 and 19 and from there to an area in the side of the brain called the parietal lobe where the image is identified. Other nerve pathways carry the message to the frontal lobe, at the front of the brain, which determines how the viewer will react to it. And there are other centers beyond this, even more intricate and less understood, which are concerned with reasoning, emotional reaction and abstract thinking. To add to this miracle, this multitude of messages, shunted through so many connections, all of them, from beginning to end, all combined, are completed in a small fraction of a second!

Considering all these intricacies, the remarkable thing is not that there are some poor readers but that there are so many good ones. For the adult good reader it may all seem very easy because he functions normally and he has been reading well for years. To get an idea of how difficult a struggle this can be for the child with dyslexia, let the adult reader try, even with the aid of a dictionary, to handle a language foreign to him, especially one printed in unfamiliar characters such as Greek, Hebrew or Chinese. Moreover, the normal adult can, with time and perseverance, ultimately learn a new language; the dyslexic usually cannot learn to read his own.

What can be done for a true dyslexic?

First, rule out all other possible causes in order to establish the diagnosis as early and as definitively as possible. This is most important because the approach depends on the correct diagnosis. If the case is one of true dyslexia, the present state of our knowledge holds out little likelihood of making the child into a good reader — but only, at best, a minimal or adequate reader.

With this prognosis in mind, the next step is to refrain from forcing the child to do what he finds impossible and frustrating. However, this must be done without recrimination and with the understanding and cooperation of all persons involved, starting of course with the parents who are the key agents.

There are some things that can be done. A program of retraining and substitute skills can steer the child in a positive way toward a satisfying and purposeful career consistent with his ability. A common compensatory education practice uses the auditory approach with recording devices and tapes in place of writing and the printed word.

Fortunately, more and more school districts are becoming aware of this problem and are making attempts to meet it. They realize that money spent on such training is returned many-fold by avoiding the wasteful expenditure of enormous sums to impart a conventional education to those who will not benefit from it.

Where can advice and help be obtained?

The actual retraining of the dyslexic child is a highly specialized procedure and does not come within the province of a book on eyes. Also it is impossible to recommend specific university reading clinics or individual teachers — since they vary so greatly in quality and availability. One must obtain the advice of the experts in the school or school district because of their knowledge of the local situation.

The U.S. Office of Education offers free advice regarding special education which may be helpful to those with learning problems, be they physical, mental or emotional. For information, write "Closer Look," Box 1492, Washington, D.C. 20013.

Obviously, the success of any program for this purpose will depend on individual variations in the children themselves, on the severity of the dyslexia — and, most important, on the skill and patience of those experts either within an institution, or in a private tutorial relationship, who are doing the retraining. It will be a comfort to parents to learn that some very important and well-known people have dyslexia, and that with devotion, concern and much hard work, their lives have been made productive and rewarding.

8
Eye Injuries: Prevention of Blindness

John Smith, aged thirty-three, was a successful salesman for a large appliance firm. He drove his car thousands of miles a year in the course of his work. His sport was tennis and his hobby was his home workshop in the basement family room. One Sunday evening, while using his power drill, he felt a sharp pain in his right eye as though a foreign object had entered it. He knew enough not to rub it and after a few minutes the pain subsided. He assumed the object had washed out. Next morning the eye was a bit sore but felt better when he bathed it with warm water. On going outdoors, he found the morning sunlight uncomfortable and put on his sunglasses. It was only when he reached the office that he found the vision in his right eye a little blurred. Because of an important business appointment, it wasn't until later that he had a chance to pay attention to his eye. In the bathroom mirror he could see no foreign object, but the eye was slightly red and he noticed that the right pupil was smaller than the left. On closing the left eye, he found the blur in the right slightly worse. Suddenly, he remembered the incident with the power drill the evening before.

That noon, in my office, examination with the ophthalmoscope (an instrument with which I look inside the pupil by sighting along a light beam) disclosed a tiny, glistening steel sliver, like the blade of a minute dagger in the back of the clear vitreous, just in front of the retina. It was, at most, an eighth of an inch long. Examination of the front of the eye with the corneal microscope showed a tiny wound in the cornea and a small perforation in the lower iris. The wound had closed so that no fluid was leaking out of the eye. Switching to the high-power lens of the instrument, I saw microscopic cells floating in the aqueous fluid — an indication that inflammation had started within the eyeball. When I dilated the pupil with drops, I found, as expected, that the tiny dagger on its way to the back of the eye had also traversed the lens, leaving a fine but unmistakable gray track through it. In so doing, it had pierced the front capsule and the back capsule of the lens. At these points clouds were just beginning to form which would, within a week, convert the entire lens into a cataract and make the eye blind.

Meanwhile Mrs. Smith, reached by telephone at home, brought the drill and bit to the office. A moment's test with an ordinary hand magnet disclosed our second piece of bad luck: the bit was non-magnetic, apparently made of one of the modern steel alloys. Therefore, the sliver within the eye, which was almost surely from this steel bit, was also non-magnetic. Had it been magnetic, the operation, while still a heroic one, would have been aided by the use of a giant magnet. In Mr. Smith's case, removal of the non-magnetic alloy splinter would unfortunately be much more difficult. The cataract which was developing in any case could, of course, wait.

Fortunately, a former student of mine, who was not only a fine ophthalmologist but also an electronic whiz, had some years earlier invented an electronic device which helps remove **non**-magnetic foreign objects from within the eyeball. That afternoon in the operating room of Manhattan Eye and Ear Hospital, he used this device to remove the steel from the inside of Mr. Smith's eye. Five weeks later, when the eye had quieted down, I removed the fully opaque cataract, restoring his vision.

Mr. Smith was one of the lucky ones. He lost only eight

weeks from work and only another eight weeks before it was safe for him to wear a cataract-contact-lens on the cured eye. He needed this contact lens to restore his binocular (two eyes at the same time) vision so that he could, after a total loss of four months, again drive a car and play tennis.

All because he didn't take three seconds to put on a pair of light, plastic protective eyeglasses or a light, one-piece protective visor before he started using his power drill!

Mr. Smith was lucky in a few other respects. Had he waited a few days instead of a few hours, had the penetrating object been larger and more blunt or dirtier, had it been copper or brass (which quickly sets up a destructive chemical inflammation inside the eyeball), had he not been able to find the steel alloy bit which was the source of the splinter (leading me to waste time operating with an ordinary giant magnet before finding that that was useless) and, most of all, had it been ten years earlier, before my young colleague had invented the non-magnetic device — in any of these circumstances he'd have fared much worse.

I have had other less fortunate patients whose injuries were much, much more severe. Some eyes were instantly destroyed beyond repair by larger and blunter flying objects. Others were so badly damaged that only partial sight could be restored — after several operations, much inconvenience, much discomfort, months in and out of hospitals and doctors' offices, and many thousands of dollars in lost salaries plus hospital and medical bills. Insurance reimbursement is small comfort and hardly a compensation for loss of sight.

And all preventable by a little protective glass or shield!

There are a great many ways to injure an eye and only two things you need to know to prevent this injury:

1. what risks to avoid and
2. how simple it is to protect your eyes when you can't avoid exposure to risk.

This chapter deals with both.

The great majority of all eye injuries are unnecessary and preventable. Ophthalmologists have known this for a long time. Unfortunately the average layman does not learn it until too late — **after** he has had an injury.

Everyone agrees on the importance of preventive medicine, but so few do anything about it. Most think that it is the job of government, that if some superagency spends enough money on it, prevention will automatically exist in sufficient abundance to do away with disease or injury. They forget that prevention starts and ends with the individual himself, that unless he participates there is no prevention. A good example: seat belts are now required by law. How many people use them?

There is hardly any other branch of medicine in which prevention is more effective than in eye injuries, and where carelessness can be so devastating. This is because the eye is so delicate, so intricate, so finely organized that even a relatively small injury can disrupt it badly and destroy its usefulness permanently.

It is my hope that you read this important chapter slowly and thoughtfully so that you may be saved from needless suffering and loss of sight. John Smith, at the head of this chapter, was of course a fictitious name. It could be yours. And you don't need a power drill. There are hundreds of other ways to get hurt, but before discussing them let me point out the single, most effective device for **preventing** the vast majority of serious eye injuries. You have already discovered it while reading about John Smith. It is the protective goggle or visor.

The importance of wearing goggles

You don't have to be a workman to wear goggles. Unfortunately, most people learn this too late — after the injury has already damaged the eye. You would not believe how often workers in hazardous industries neglect wearing their goggles. The following dialogue takes place routinely while I am treating one of them who has had an eye injury. The questions and answers hardly ever vary:

> "Don't you have goggles where you work?"
> "Sure."
> "Why didn't you wear them?"
> "Doc, I can't see with them."
> My invariable reply: "Better than with a glass eye."
> "Yeah, that's for sure."

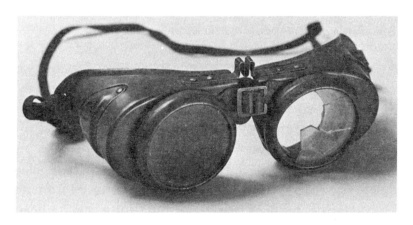

Fig. 6. This pair of safety goggles was brought to me by a patient after he had been in an accident at work. Some of the safety glass, broken by a flying piece of steel, hit his eye. But the goggles saved his sight, and probably his life.

I then take down a shattered goggle which hangs on the wall of my treatment room. I describe the trivial nature of the injury sustained by the wearer and, for comparison, the total disaster in a similar accident without this protection. They always promise me never again to handle a power tool without safety glasses. Some of them keep that promise.

You don't have to be working for a boss to wear protective lenses. The metal particle flying toward your eye with the speed of a bullet doesn't know that you are only a hobbyist with an electric drill. This is proven by the striking increase of serious eye injuries among the growing army of do-it-yourselfers — the users of home workshops, high speed electrical tools:

> drills
> saws
> chisels
> solderers
> sanders
> polishers
> mowers
> cutters
> sprayers
> chain-saws.

In two senses the hobbyist is even worse off than the workman: (1) the latter's boss can insist that goggles be worn, a power not vested in the hobbyist's spouse, (2) the injured employee's medical, hospital and living expenses are paid by workmen's compensation insurance. Many a hobbyist without personal accident insurance has been made bankrupt by medical and hospital expenses at the very time when his salary was stopped because he was unable to work.

Inflexible rule: Never use any motor driven tool without protecting the eyes. The same holds true for any hand tool where there is any chance of a flying particle. Goggles or visors are also excellent protections when handling chemicals such as industrial acids, battery acids, battery jump cables [batteries explode, scattering acid], paint thinners and removers, strong detergents or bleaches, lye for cleaning home drains, and soldering or plastering materials.

Protection need not be by heavy welder's goggles. A simple one-piece clear plastic visor, easily obtainable in most opticians' shops, hobby shops, pharmacies, will give fair protection against most flying particles. These visors are surprisingly light, can be worn with a headband or with ear pieces like spectacles, or clipped on to one's own spectacles.

If you wear ordinary glasses and you obtained your last pair since January 1, 1972, you are probably protected because, since that date all spectacle lenses are, by federal law, safety glasses, i.e., plastic or shatterproof glass. To be certain, ask the optician who made them.

At this point it is appropriate to mention a national organization which has pioneered for eye safety and which has been the greatest single force in the campaign to popularize protective lenses, the National Society for the Prevention of Blindness. Its constant publicity in industrial plants, schools, and laboratories directed toward employees, managers, doctors, students and the general public has unquestionably prevented many thousands of eye injuries, untold disability and suffering, and has saved many many millions of dollars for the public. All this has been done at no cost to the public or to the government because this splendid work is supported entirely by voluntary contributions. I'm sure I speak for all eye specialists when I express gratitude for what this organization continually does to protect our patients and incidentally lighten our work load. The National Society for the Prevention of Blindness surely deserves the voluntary financial support of everyone who considers eyesight precious.

WHAT TO DO FOR EYE INJURIES

Second in importance to prevention is some knowledge of what to do when there is an eye injury; also what **not** to do depending on the nature of the injury.

There is of course no substitute (in any but the most minor mishaps) for getting the patient to an eye specialist if one is easily available.

Chemical injuries are different

But before proceeding, and while your attention is at its peak, I am going to make one important exception to this rule:

Do **not** start looking for an eye specialist if a **chemical** gets into the eye.

You are wasting precious seconds! Every second that a chemical remains in the eye without being immediately washed out increases the amount of damage which may well be permanent. Seconds count — not minutes, but seconds. Run, do not walk, to the nearest source of water and gently but liberally let it flow into the eye, washing out or at least diluting the chemical. The ideal sink is in the kitchen rather than the bathroom because the faucet in the kitchen is high enough so that, with a little contortion, the patient can be placed **under** it, face up, to let a **gentle** stream of cool water run directly into the eye. The eye must be forcibly held open by the patient's own thumb and forefinger. If such a faucet is not instantly available, it is better **immediately** to take water from any source in the cupped hand and splash it repeatedly into the open eye. Then if a cup, tumbler or kettle with a spout is available, gently pour cool water from any of these vessels repeatedly into the open eye for a couple of minutes.

Do **not** waste time doing the following:
1. Do **not** telephone the doctor. (Of course you will do this **after** you have washed the eye.)
2. Do **not** look for an eye cup.
3. Do **not** look for Boric Acid.
4. Do **not** boil the water.
5. Do **not** fuss about protecting your clothes from getting wet at the sink.

After washing the eye, do not rub it while drying your face. Gently pat the closed eye with a towel until dry. **Then** telephone the eye specialist. Unless there is much pain, do not patch the eye; the tearing of the open eye is beneficial because tears are antiseptic and also help to wash out any remaining chemical. After fifteen minutes or so, if there is pain, you may then patch the eye especially if it will be some time before you can see the specialist. Do **not** put salve into the eye. **Do** save the box or bottle of the offending chemical, together with its label, and bring it to the eye specialist so that he may determine the nature of the chemical more precisely.

I have gone into great detail and discussed this first because chemical burn is the only kind of eye injury in which seconds count. What you do, and how quickly, can be literally 95% of the battle for sight.

One more thing: What do we mean by "chemical"? Anything which reacts with or irritates the surface of the eyeball, the cornea, or the lining of the eyelid and thus causes the cornea to become cloudy. Here is a partial list of the most common substances to which the eye is subject — in factory, shop, home, school or laboratory:

Acids: hydrochloric (muriatic), sulphuric, nitric used in industry. Battery acids.

Alkalis, especially sodium and potassium, also used in industry. Lye, used in the home to clean drains is a frequent and powerful offender, as is lime used in building and repairing.

Solvents, gasoline, kerosene, benzine, carbon tetrachloride, antifreeze, cleaning fluids, paint thinners, paint removers, alcohol, ether.

Concentrated detergents
Bleaches
Hair sprays
Insect sprays
Plant sprays
Oven cleansers
Adhesive fluids
Glues
Solders

I'm sure by now I need not point out to you that practically every one of the chemicals mentioned can be kept out of the eye by scrupulously wearing protective glasses or visors whenever handling any of them, be it in factory, shop, school, laboratory or home — including hobby workshop.

"MINOR" EYE INJURIES

The word "minor" is only relative because there are really no **minor** eye injuries. With an organ so delicate, any small injury can become a major catastrophe. However, compared to chemical burns and perforations, they are less disastrous.

The black eye

To the boy who has been fighting or playing football, a black eye is just a "shiner." Usually it is only that and it goes away in a week or so.

But a small percentage of black eyes are more serious. Any blow severe enough to cause a "shiner" — a hemorrhage under the skin of the eyelid — may also injure the eye itself. Fortunately this is rare because the eyeball is partly protected by the bones of the socket, the brow above and the cheek below, plus the fatty padding all around the eye as it lies within the socket.

But if the eyeball itself sustains part of the blow, certain complications are possible. The most common of these are: torn retina — leading to detachment, torn choroid, dislocation of the lens, iritis (an inflammation of the iris), hemorrhage within the eyeball. All of these are serious and a threat to the sight, even if treated — more so if not treated, or treated too late. With a more severe blow there is also the possibility of a fracture of the bone of the socket.

How do you judge? Usually you can't. And if every boy with a "shiner" were to be rushed for examination, there would not be enough ophthalmologists. There is, however, one criterion you can use, and that is the effect on the sight. In the ordinary black eye the vision is not blurred, although even in these, detachments have occurred later. But if, on covering the opposite eye, the sight of the affected eye is impaired, it means that the eyeball has been struck and an eye specialist should examine it without great delay. The same is true if, with both eyes open, there is double vision which may be an indication of fracture of the bone of the socket.

Foreign objects

This is the most common minor injury and if properly attended rarely causes serious or permanent damage. Most foreign objects are blown or shaken in and many will come out by themselves. The best immediate treatment is to keep your hands away from your eyes (to avoid rubbing) and continually to blink the lids. The mechanical action of blinking plus the flow of tears will wash most objects out. If the object is lodged on the surface of the cornea, rubbing merely presses it into the cornea so that it becomes embedded. If it does not wash out after a few minutes, try rolling the eyes about while opening and closing the lids. Then grasp the lashes and pull the upper lid gently downward and a little away from the eyeball. Some persons are able to evert (turn over) the upper lid; a foreign object found on the lid's under-surface may be lightly dislodged with a clean applicator.

If the object is embedded in the surface of the cornea the situation is quite different, especially if a careful search under good light, with a magnifying lens or in a magnifying mirror, discloses that the object is in the **center** of the cornea, in front of the black pupil. Such an object is best removed by an eye specialist because, if not done properly, a tiny scar is left in the pupillary area which may affect the sight. The specialist anesthetizes the cornea with a few drops so that there is absolutely no sensation or pain when the object is removed. He uses a fine instrument, under the magnification of the corneal microscope, so that he does not touch the cornea and damage it. And he usually patches the eye for at least a day to encourage the tiny crater to heal.

Strangely — and this is one of nature's 'mistakes' — a foreign object lodged in the lining of the **upper eyelid** where it can do relatively little harm is so extremely painful (because with each blink it scrapes the exquisitely sensitive cornea) that the patient runs for help right away. By contrast, an object which is embedded in the surface of the **cornea** where its continued presence can cause serious inflammation and even scarring, will for the first few days be only slightly painful (because it is stationary in the cornea; with eye movement it rubs only against the lining of the upper lid which is relatively insensitive). During those few days the eye may feel only slightly scratchy, it may tear and be a little sensitive to light — sometimes so little that it is easy to ignore. It may be only after a few days have passed, when the continued presence of the object, embedded in the surface of the cornea, has brought on an inflammation, that the pain of that inflammation sends the patient to the doctor. By then, the situation may be serious.

The lesson from this? If an eye feels suddenly slightly irritated, teary and sensitive to light, try looking at the surface of the cornea under good light, if possible using a magnifier. If there is an object lodged there, do not try to pick it off yourself because your manipulation may scratch the cornea and do more harm to the delicate surface than would the foreign object. Get to an eye specialist, eye clinic or eye hospital emergency room. Even though you have been unable to detect a foreign object, if the symptoms persist for one more day, you should seek help.

Abrasion of the cornea

This is a common superficial injury in which the front surface of the cornea is scratched. Depending on the extent of the area scraped off, the pain may be slight or severe and may persist for a few hours to days or weeks, until the abrasion is healed. It occurs most frequently in mothers whose eyes are scratched by their infants' untrimmed fingernails, but it can be inflicted on anyone by an adult's nails, by the corner of a magazine or theater program, by a towel, sheet, brush, comb, mascara brush, eyebrow tweezers, kitchen utensils, drapes, twigs, tools, and of course in industry. Abrasions may be caused by contact lenses: by carelessness in insertion or removal, or if they are faulty, irregular or rough; also if wearers forget to remove them before going to sleep, or if they fail to remove them whenever a foreign object lodges in the eye underneath the contact lens.

The pain of a scratched cornea may not become severe until an hour or more has elapsed, but by the next morning the patient is at the ophthalmologist's office in agony, having been kept awake all night. He swears that the eye feels as though it is full of sand and is worse if he moves the eye or tries to open or close it.

The eye specialist puts into the eye a minute amount of vegetable dye called fluorescein which shows up the denuded portion of the cornea by staining it bright green, in contrast to the uninjured part of the cornea which does not stain. Daily staining enables him to tell the progress of healing as the staining area becomes smaller and smaller. If, with rest, patching, sedation and anitseptics, the area can be made to heal without infection, it will usually leave no scar.

The most important part of the treatment is rest, to allow the injured corneal surface, protected by the closed, patched eyelid, to heal as rapidly and as cleanly as possible. Patching alone without rest is not sufficient because if the opposite eye is in use, its movements will also cause the injured eye to move and delay the healing. I usually send these patients home to bed with enough sedation to allow them to sleep soundly. In a few days most eyes are healed and free of pain and may resume normal activity.

When healed, the patient must be warned against rubbing that eye for the next few months because of the possibility of an annoying complication: recurrent erosion.

Recurrent erosion of an injured cornea

Recurrent erosion is the repeated breakdown of the healed abrasion causing repeated attacks of pain similar to that of the original injury. Its natural history is as follows:

A person suffers an abrasion of the cornea as just described. Healing takes place after a number of days but the newly healed area is never as firm as it was before the injury. It may be even less firm if the eye was not sufficiently at rest during the healing process, if there was lowered resistance or poor healing capacity, if the bandage was removed too soon, if activity was resumed too soon, or merely just because of bad luck.

One morning, any time from a few days to a few months after the injury, the patient awakens with a sharp stabbing pain in the eye as severe as that of the original injury. What has happened is a loosening of the healed surface, possibly because he rubbed his eye during sleep, possibly because the overlying closed lid, touching the cornea all night, pulls on the corneal surface at the instant the eyelids are opened. This is most common when a crying infant awakens a parent at night: the quick, sudden opening of the eyes causes a sharp, severe pain in the formerly injured eye. This usually requires treatment and patching for a few hours to a few days.

Worse still, a pattern of recurrent erosion, once established, usually leads to further recurrences, much annoyance, disability and expense. Conversely, the longer the cornea goes without a recurrent erosion, the less likely it is to get one.

The best treatment is prevention. I warn patients to avoid rubbing the eye for at least several months after an abrasion. If there are recurrences, I prescribe a bland lubricant for the eye at bedtime and the wearing of an aluminum eye shield during sleep, similar to that worn after cataract operation, to keep the eyes from being rubbed by the fingers or by the pillow. I also caution the patient to avoid opening the eyes abruptly on awakening, but rather to lie awake with the eyes closed for a few seconds before opening them **slowly**.

If, despite these precautions, the erosions are persistent, frequent and disabling, I gently remove the entire damaged corneal surface so that it has a chance to heal afresh and more firmly. This is a minor operation, painless under local anesthesia, performed with the aid of a corneal microscope for greater precision. The eye is then patched for a few days while the patient remains at rest under mild sedation. It usually cures the condition.

Sun lamp burn, welding flash, snow blindness

These are all ultraviolet light burns of the cornea and of the surface of the eyeball. They can all be frighteningly painful, made worse by their sudden onset 6 to 9 hours **after** the exposure, sometimes in the middle of the night, long enough for the exposure to have been forgotten. The patient feels as though there are a thousand particles of sand in each eye and when he tries to look at the eyes, the light causes excruciating pain. Treatment by an eye specialist need be only for relief of discomfort. The condition subsides in two to five days, leaving no permanent damage, but the patient is a bit shaken by the experience.

I remember years ago, a colleague and long-time friend, a dermatologist, telephoned me at 2 A.M. shouting into the phone, "Ben, I'm blind, both eyes, full of sand, the light is killing me!" I answered: "Before you say anymore, tell me — did you manage to fix your ultra-violet sun lamp last night?" "Oh! My goodness," he exclaimed, "I had forgotten! How did you know?" I answered: "It's now 2 A.M.; your office hours are over at 6 and you must have tinkered with your sun lamp after dinner, about seven hours ago. Because it was not a treatment, you forgot that you needed to put on your own goggles." "Exactly right. What a relief. And I thought I was going blind." Three days later he was back at work.

Strangely, one need not even wear goggles when getting a sun lamp treatment. One need only remember that the eyes should be closed before the switch is turned on and **not** opened again until the current has been turned off. Ultraviolet rays will not go through the eyelids; they will cause a slight burn of the skin of the eyelids along with the rest of the face.

Welding flash works the same way with one difference: the ultraviolet rays are delivered to the eyes in one large dose, sometimes in a fraction of a second, instead of weaker doses over a few minutes (sun lamp) or over a few hours (snow blindness). Such a burn is rarely sustained by welders who know how to protect themselves while working, but it occurs among bystanders or those who work **near** welders who think they are too far away to need protection. It also occurs among electricians who inadvertently set off an electric arc and are not wearing protective glasses while working.

Why do skiers without goggles become snow blind while people on a tropical beach become sunburned but not snow blind? Because sunbathers get most of their ultraviolet rays from above. The cornea is protected to some extent by the brow, upper lid and eyelashes; skiers get their exposure to light rays as much from **below** by reflection from the snow as they do directly from the sun above.

Eclipse blindness

This condition is in **no** way related to snow blindness. Unlike the latter, eclipse blindness is very serious and often results in **permanent** damage to the center of vision, impairing the ability to read and barring a person from many kinds of jobs which require good vision.

This damage is caused by prolonged exposure of the macula to the sun while the eye continues to fix its gaze directly on it just before and after the eclipse. Normally the sun, even on a cloudy day, is so bright that it is impossible to focus directly on it for more than a second. Just before and after the eclipse, the sun's light is sufficiently reduced so that viewers focus on it with little or no discomfort. It is the **prolonged** exposure of the one spot, rather than the intensity, which does the damage.

This catastrophe befalls a great many people after each eclipse. It happens even if they take the precaution of watching through sun glasses or photographic film. It can be prevented by watching for not more than a few seconds or by viewing only a reflection from the surface of a still pond or of water in a vessel. Water absorbs much of the light rays. However, do not use a mirror for it does reflect most of the light.

Concentrated detergents

Many strong cleansers and bleaches are, for reasons of economy, purchased in high concentrations and used in small amounts highly diluted in water. Housewives and industrial workers may accidentally splash the concentrated fluid into the eyes before or during the mixing. This is particularly true of those detergents labelled "gentle" in the ads. These "gentle" chemicals, when they come out of the bottle in their pure, concentrated form, are strong enough to burn the surface of the cornea. So, **before** you dilute them, handle them with care. It is only **after** they are highly diluted — a few drops in a pan of water — that they are harmless and "gentle."

Rarely, children or childish adults playfully squirt some of this concentrate into a friend's face, thinking it is harmless — with drastic results.

When mixing strong chemicals, prevent injury by wearing glasses during the mixing process. If the eye is splashed, treat like any other chemical burn, instantly pouring cool water into the open eye. If the offending substance is a detergent, follow this up by bathing the open eye with **milk** — ordinary milk from the refrigerator — which partially neutralizes some detergent concentrates.

Lesser irritants; sprays

Some substances are irritating to the eyes but in normal strengths rarely cause permanent damage. These include the various aerosol sprays such as hair fixatives, deodorants, plant sprays, paint sprays, various cleansers (oven, bathroom, window). Most aerosol sprays contain a compressed gas (Freon) which, when released by the trigger on the can, expands to act as the propellant of the active chemical. This is ejected with considerable force, especially when the can is new or warm. Such a blast, wrongly aimed, striking an open eye, can cause great pain.

In addition, there are increasing reports of microscopic particles of the spray being blown with such force that they penetrate **under** the surface of the cornea to lodge permanently within its thickness. These rarely affect the sight but may be a permanent source of irritation, discomfort and tearing.

Lesson: When using a spray can, make sure the arrow on the valve points **away** from you. If it's a hair spray, or any cosmetic, take the added precaution of keeping the eyes closed during the actual spraying. When spraying stronger chemicals, like oven cleaner or spray detergents, it is best to wear glasses.

Chlorinated swimming pools

The chlorine in pools is so highly diluted as to be harmless to the eyes, although swimmers report some irritation and redness for an hour or two after leaving the pool. Swimming is one of the world's best exercises and recreations, and it would be only under very special circumstances that I would advise abstaining merely to avoid the chlorinated water.

There is another condition which occasionally troubles those who swim for long periods in **fresh** water — a temporary faint haziness of vision sometimes accompanied by slight discomfort, tearing and sensitivity to light. It is caused by the prolonged contact (soaking) of the surface of the cornea with the **fresh** water, especially after extended periods underwater as in scuba diving without goggles or mask. This never happens in salt water (sea water) because the salt concentration in sea water is the same as that in tears and in the fluids within the cornea. Fresh water, with no significant salt content, tends to be absorbed in minute amounts into the corneal surface, causing faint swelling and haziness of vision. This disappears within a half hour after coming out of the water. It is usually harmless, though annoying, and can be minimized by closing the eyes occasionally during prolonged swimming, or if scuba diving in **fresh** water, by wearing goggles.

The more destructive eye injuries
Contusions and perforations

These are the most serious of the eye injuries, involving, as they do, the potential for blindness.

A contusion is a blow with a blunt object; a perforation usually is caused by a sharp object penetrating into the interior of the eyeball. Sometimes the blunt object strikes with enough force to burst the eyeball, in which case the distinction between contusion and perforation becomes irrelevant. Either one, if more than slight, is a major catastrophe.

What to do is relatively simple: Get medical attention, preferably that of an eye specialist, as soon as reasonably possible and in the interim keep the patient fairly quiet. If you are the injured person, try to get someone to act for you so that you yourself can remain reasonably quiet.

What **NOT** to do is equally important: Do not do anything to make the injured eye worse. This means:

Do NOT panic. Remain as calm as possible in a difficult situation. Most people panic not only because of the calamity, but because they feel lost, helpless and frustrated in not really knowing how to act. One of the reasons for this chapter is to fortify you **in advance** so that you know how to act if ever necessary — a kind of mental fire-drill.

Furthermore, I have added the **reason** for each of the following commandments. If you understand why, you will remember them better and do less harm.

Do NOT wash the injured eye. There is nothing gained by washing, even if the object which struck the eye is dirty. (Remember — this rule is not valid if a chemical liquid or powder has splashed into the eye. These must be washed out at once.) You cannot get **all** the dirty material out; you cannot sterilize the area no matter how hard you try. And if the eye is indeed perforated you can do an incalculable amount of damage, not only by introducing fluids but also by disrupting the eyeball with manipulation and involuntary squeezing of the eyelids. I have seen many perforated injuries made very much worse by the struggle to wash the eye — which resulted in some or all of the ocular contents being extruded through the wound.

By the same token, don't waste time looking for boric acid or an eye cup or boiling the water. Stay away from the eye.

Do NOT put salves or any medicines in the injured eye. No matter how much of a believer you are in potent antibiotics. The reasons against this are same as for not washing. In addition, salve inside a perforation can do much more harm than good.

Do NOT remove any blood or bloodclots from the eye. It is all right to sponge off the face, but keep away from the eye. Don't worry about the appearance or the bloody clothes. Don't worry about loss of blood; in the many hundreds of eye injuries I have treated, I have never once seen enough blood lost from an eye alone to even consider a transfusion. Besides, blood contains antiseptics which are good for the injured tissue.

I remember one evening treating a young man whose eye had been cut when his eyeglasses were broken in a high school basketball game. The person accompanying him knew just enough about first aid to make him dangerous. He proudly described to me how he had washed the eye and removed the blood clot. The clot was the iris!

Do NOT try to force the eyelids open to look at the eye if the patient cannot open it easily by himself. Even if he can, but doing so makes him wince and squeeze involuntarily because of pain or sensitivity to light — leave him alone.

Do NOT march the patient about unnecessarily if a place to lie down is readily available. This does not mean that he cannot be walked to get indoors, or up a flight of stairs or to a bed, car or ambulance, if necessary. But the less walking the better. And do not let him walk unaided, especially on stairs. Remember that a person suddenly reduced to seeing with only one eye is unable to judge distance, and could fall down stairs, or while getting in and out of a car. I have seen eyes badly injured a second time in this way.

Also, although the injured eye is closed or bandaged, the use of the **un**injured eye should be limited because the two eyes move together, as a team; and moving one eye causes the other to move.

Do NOT waste time looking for or buying a special eye patch. Any clean cloth such as a clean folded handkerchief will do. It can be attached with **slight** firmness over the closed eye with adhesive or scotch tape to forehead and cheek. If the face is too bloody or wet for tape, a light bandage will hold it. The patch need not be sterile, merely clean. The skin of your eyelid isn't sterile.

Do NOT feed the patient before going to the doctor. It is important that the stomach be as empty as possible because, if emergency surgery has to be done under general anesthesia, food in the stomach can delay matters and make anesthesia more difficult and hazardous.

This is especially true in the case of children who would probably require a general anesthetic. But too often an injured child's mother makes sure to feed him, lest he starve before he reaches the hospital or arrives after mealtime.

Anesthetists rightly dread administering a general anesthetic when there is food in the stomach because of the danger of serious complications and even of death if retained food is regurgitated by the semi-conscious patient, and then gets breathed into the lungs. For this reason, they correctly insist upon delaying the operation a few hours or until next morning if the patient has just had a full meal. Rarely does a few hours' delay make a substantial difference to the outcome. With injuries to other more remote parts of the body, one can avoid this delay by passing a stomach tube and pumping out the stomach contents. But after an eye injury, this is highly undesirable because the retching and vomiting induced by the tube could aggravate the injury. Also, even if no surgery is necessary, a recent meal in a patient, who is frightened or in pain, may in itself be a cause of nausea or vomiting — which is bad for the injured eye.

On the other hand, there is no objection to drinking water, in small quantities, as much or as often as desired, plus a little fruit juice, but not milk. There is an advantage, especially with children, in not being too dehydrated.

And finally, I repeat the first admonition: **Don't panic**. Panic is quickly contagious and easily transmitted, especially to children. It makes everything more difficult — the waiting, the much needed calm while waiting, the examination, the treatment, the induction of anesthesia and even the post-operative period of convalescence — all can be more stormy and therefore more hazardous because of the patient's emotional state. In fact, it is not unusual for the doctor to suggest during the telephone conversation that the patient take a mild tranquillizer before coming to the office.

Getting the doctor

This also involves some **DOs and DON'Ts**.

Telephone your doctor reasonably soon after you have evaluated the situation.

Do NOT wait to phone until after the arrival of your spouse, the children, or someone who can drive. The doctor you want may be immediately available at the moment but out of reach if you delay calling until later, and the answering service has to trace him or a substitute.

Do NOT try to save time by dashing to the doctor's office. He may not be there. Save time by using the telephone. If he is not there, the nurse or the answering service or even the recorded message will tell you where he is or what to do. If the line is continually busy, the chief operator will, if you explain the emergency to her, cut in to get your number.

Once connected, DON'T hang up if you get an answering service or a taped message, and don't insist on speaking to no one but the doctor. Simply say clearly: "This is an emergency. I have just had an eye injury." (And, if it's true: "I can't see with the eye," or "My vision is blurred.") Then listen and follow instructions. The nurse or receptionist or answering service is there to help you and is carefully trained to act properly and promptly in such a situation. Don't try to take charge and run the show — you only interfere with what would normally be a smooth routine.

If the doctor will be unavailable for too long and a substitute is not suggested, ask for one.

If the response is by a tape recorded message, **DON'T hang up** but listen. It will tell you what to do.

Another friend in need is your family doctor or pediatrician or internist — and you **should** have one, in any event, who knows you. Although he will probably prefer not to treat the eye injury, he is available to find you an eye specialist if you can't; and if you have a specialist he will probably want to consult with him about your medical status, drug idiosyncracies, immunizations, etc.

In the remote chance that you have still gotten nowhere, there are two other possibilities for finding an eye specialist: the local medical society and the local hospital. Most counties have an emergency telephone number in the Yellow Pages at the head of "Physicians and Surgeons." It is usually the number of the local county medical society where you will obtain a list of eye specialists in your vicinity. The local hospital will do the same. If the hospital telephone operator cannot help you, ask her to connect you with the person in charge of the emergency room. If she can refer you to an available eye specialist on their staff to see you in the emergency room or in his office, that is preferable to being treated by general emergency room personnel — who are usually very competent but who may not have been trained in eye work (and will probably end up by sending you to an eye specialist anyway). The exception to this is in larger cities where there may be an **eye** hospital; at such institutions the emergency room personnel **is** trained in eye work.

If possible, avoid long, jolting trips to a distant specialist if a nearby specialist is not instantly available. A wait of an hour or two will not usually make much difference once the damage has been done. However, the patient should be kept reasonably quiet or even sedated while waiting.

You have telephoned the doctor and have been told when to come to the office. Remember: No food. If you are the patient and alone, it is best not to walk or to drive yourself. Take a taxi or let a neighbor drive you. If the patient is a child and both parents are available, it is best for **both** to come, but leave the other children at home or in the care of a neighbor. Small children tagging along, demanding attention, are what you and the doctor do **not** need in an emergency situation.

Once in the eye specialist's hands you have nothing more to do but be the patient. From that point, all decisions and actions are his. But remember, no matter how great his skill, the damage to the eye was probably established at the moment of the injury. You may be encouraged by the assurance that, as a certified eye specialist, he became one only after many years of meticulous training, and therefore the chance of saving the eye is excellent if it has not been damaged beyond repair.

The removal of an injured eye

With the steady and dramatic improvement in all aspects of treatment and surgery, an ever greater percentage of injured eyes is being saved. However, there will always be an irreducible minimum of eyes so badly damaged that the ultimate grim fate of removal is unavoidable.

Contrary to some popular hopes, the complete transplant (replacement) of a whole eye is still out of the question and will be for the near future. Corneas, lenses and even vitreous can now routinely be replaced, wounds meticulously repaired, and retinas reattached, but occasionally an eye which has been severely disrupted by injury and derangement of its delicate internal components will remain blind despite all efforts at cure.

This alone does not call for removal of the eye, but other developments might. They are: intractable pain, severe disfigurement, and above all, the danger in certain cases of sympathetic inflammation of the opposite eye — in other words the spectre of complete blindness of both eyes. Faced with this, one has practically no alternative but to recommend removal, and foolhardy would be the patient or family to disagree. In such a tragic pass, it is but slight consolation for the victim to tell him that, although he is naturally against removing the eye, he is really losing nothing because there is no chance that it will ever see again.

The new artificial eye will be free of pain, will not be ugly but will look like a normal eye, and will not see any less than the blinded one. The operation will be painless under either local anesthesia or general anesthesia, he will be out of bed the next day and out of the hospital in a few days. Best of all, he may have eliminated the danger to his remaining good eye with which he can carry on almost normally for the rest of his life. (See Chapter 10 on one-eyed vision.)

Today's artificial eye is natural looking and not disfiguring. Made by highly skilled artisans out of plastic and acryllic rather than glass, it is matched perfectly to the other eye. In the removal surgery, the eye muscles are now retained so that the new eye moves in sufficient coordination with the other eye to give the illusion that both are seeing together. In fact they look so normal that, in most cases before operating, I advise the patient and the family to avoid publicizing the prospective removal, so that those outside the family are not aware of it. This saves the patient the embarrassment of having friends covertly sneaking glances to see which eye is the artificial one. I have playfully fooled more than a few medical students by assigning them the examination of such eyes. Some reported that the pupil failed to contract when exposed to a bright light; others, feeling it with the fingertips through the closed eyelid, diagnosed a "hard" eye, probably a glaucoma. The patient enjoyed being part of the prank and was vastly reassured because his camouflage had deceived a medical student.

Some injuries cannot be prevented; some can

Although goggles or plastic shields are an absolute "must" in industry and hobbies, not all eye injuries occur in the course of these pursuits. Because people just don't go about wearing protective goggles, there is some unavoidable exposure in the mere act of living. Injuries may be caused by:

Protruding objects: blunt or sharp

Thrown objects: accidentally, playfully or in anger
Wielded objects: sticks, knives, fists
Ball sports: baseball, tennis, handball,
    squash, hockey
Contact sports: boxing, wrestling, water polo
Automobile accidents, broken windshields
The exploding matchhead, struck in damp weather.

On the other hand, there are certain hazards which are avoidable; indulging in them is so obviously looking for trouble that one would think warnings superfluous. They are

Fireworks
Firecrackers
Firearms, without careful instruction in their use
Air-rifles — illegal for children in most states
Slingshots
Bows-and-arrows
Duelling without face masks
Gas explosions during search for a gas leak
Exploding auto batteries
Use of high speed tools without goggles.

Other, less obvious hazards are worth a warning. Although rarer, they can be very destructive when they do happen:

Eye injuries from broken, worn-out or improperly wielded tools. The classic example is the splayed steel chisel struck by a steel hammer. Bits of the chisel fly off and penetrate the eyeball. Lesson: Never use a steel hammer on a steel chisel. Use a wooden or leaden mallet or wear a goggle or shield. Another example is the springing nail: badly struck while nailing a board which is not firm but vibrates, the nail springs back and pierces the eye. Lesson: Unless the wood is soft or solid, wear a goggle.

The popping champagne cork is expelled from the bottle with great force. It has destroyed many an eye on New Year's eve. Lesson: When opening a bottle of champagne or bubbly wine, always wrap the cork end in a towel first. Never bend over it or point it in anyone's direction, not even your own.

The fishhook, caught in the eye of a friend or bystander. The hook, whipped through the air with tremendous speed, has been known to slice an eyeball in half. Lesson: Stay more than a rod's length away from anyone casting.

And, last but not least, there is the misread or absent label:

Miss Jane Johnson, 24, was a beautiful and talented actress. At the intermission of one performance, her eyes were sandy and heavy with fatigue. She went to her dressing table and used drops to freshen her eyes. She never got to the second eye but ran screaming all over the backstage area. Had she stopped long enough to pour water immediately into the eye, it might have been saved. A half hour later, at the eye hospital, her cornea was as white and opaque as a sheet of paper. After six weeks struggle and pain, a corneal graft was done and vision restored.

Miss Johnson had been too tired and keyed up to spend an instant examining the label on the "eye drop" bottle. She used, by mistake, another dropper bottle containing concentrated creosote, which she normally diluted a thousand times (one drop to a glass of water as a gargle for clearing her voice before a performance).

Lesson: Never use an eye drop (or any medication) without first examining the label — no matter how many times a day you do so, no matter how familiar the container. Our nurses are trained, from student days, to examine the label **three** times: once when they take out the bottle, once again before they put in the drop and a third time, after instilling the drop, before returning the bottle to its tray.

One other precaution: it has become fashionable among pharmacists to dispense eye medicine bottles inside another plastic vial for the sake of cleanliness. This plastic vial protects the bottle with its dropper or cap, especially when it is carried in purse or pocket. Sometimes the pharmacist pastes the label on this outside vial rather than on the bottle itself. This is unacceptable and dangerous because the outside vial can be lost or changed. The label should be firmly fixed to the dropper bottle or squeeze bottle **itself**. If it is not, ask the pharmacist to do so and if he objects, show him the story of Miss Johnson.

Note: What is blindness?

Blindness is absence of sight. It varies in extent from one afflicted individual to another. When most profound, there is no perception of light (usually hopeless and permanent). If less severe, hand movements may be distinguished or even fingers counted a few yards away. Such a person might walk about unaided in safe territory but not cross roadways. Still better is acuity of 20/200 (see chart, p. 14) which may allow reading newspaper headlines.

Legal definitions of blindness vary from state to state. The only uniform one is the federal standard for an additional tax exemption: 20/200 with best possible correction (glass) in the better eye or side vision no wider than 20 degrees. (A certificate from the taxpayer's doctor is required.)

9
The Inflamed Eye

WARNING — Reading this chapter can be hazardous to your health — if the little you learn tempts you to treat an inflamed eye, yourself. This chapter, like all the others, is for information only. It is not a do-it-yourself guide. Treatment should be by your medical doctor or by your medical eye specialist. No one else has the knowledge — not the pharmacist, nor the optometrist, nor the nurse in plant or school. Every eye specialist has seen sick eyes needlessly damaged because the patient wasted valuable time with soothing eye drops or boric acid eye washes when vigorous treatment should have been given promptly. "I thought it was just a cold and I bathed it with boric acid" — by the time a patient comes to me with this sad story, it is often too late to help.

By contrast, not all inflamed eyes are dangerous. Some are only ugly and a bit uncomfortable. Some of the ugliest looking conditions can be the most harmless, and they often clear up without treatment. Here again, only the doctor can tell.

The blood spot

Before discussing the kinds of red eye and some of their causes, let me describe one which is the most frightening and at the same time the most innocuous — the blood spot on the white of the eye, technically known as a "sub-conjunctival hemorrhage." It is bright red because it is, in fact, fresh blood and it looks even brighter on the white background. It may be as small as a pinhead or large enough to cover the entire white and it may even contain a slightly raised clot or two. There is no blurring of vision, no discharge and no pain. In fact, so little does the patient feel, that he may be unaware of anything wrong until he happens to see the eye in the mirror or until someone calls it to his attention. In a panic, he rushes to the specialist who examines the eye to make sure nothing else is wrong, and reassures him that the spot will fade away within a week or two without treatment.

Such a hemorrhage is a drop of blood which has leaked from a break in one of the tiny blood vessels on the surface of the eyeball. It spreads out in the space between the sclera (the white of the eye) and the conjunctiva (the thin transparent membrane which covers the sclera). Because it is **under** the conjunctiva (subconjunctival) it does not wash away with the tears or with an eye wash, but gradually absorbs.

Why does the tiny vessel break? The cause may not be apparent. It frequently happens in healthy patients with normal eyes. It is more common in older persons whose blood vessels are a little more brittle, especially in those who are overweight, whose blood pressure is above normal, or who have diabetes, anemia or hardening of the arteries. It may follow an injury, or heavy lifting or straining — as in violent coughing, sneezing, retching or in straining during a bowel movement. Or, to repeat, it may be caused by none of these. The specialist may suggest a medical checkup if this has not been done within the year. Repeated hemorrhages certainly do call for such a checkup.

The bloodshot eye

It is easy to distinguish between the bloodshot eye and the harmless hemorrhage we have just described. The hemorrhage is a uniformly bright red blotch which looks like a spread-out drop of blood. The bloodshot eye, by contrast, is reddish or pinkish because the dozens of tiny blood vessels on the white — normally not noticeable — have become very swollen and therefore visible. If your eye is bloodshot, look at it carefully in a mirror (a magnifying mirror if you are over 45) and you will see the tiny, individual, swollen red blood vessels which have turned the white eye pink. Compare these vessels with the almost invisible ones on the white of your other eye or on someone else's normal eye.

There are many kinds of bloodshot eyes, but only the doctor can distinguish the serious from the trivial.

Fortunately, the ordinary reddish eye of the "morning-after" variety, or that caused by exposure to smoke, smog, dust, or fatigue has its own interesting mechanism for curing itself — the tear fluid.

Patients often ask: "Should I bathe my eye?" "Should I use an eye-wash?" "Should I use Boric Acid?" "Should I use an eye-cup?" "Should I use eye drops regularly?" The answer is, "No." Bathing is of little value medically except for mechanical cleansing of accumulated pus or crusts: it is otherwise unnecessary unless specifically ordered by the doctor, for the purpose of applying heat or cold. The eye has its own eye-wash — the tear fluid — much superior to anything you can use, short of an antibiotic or other prescription drop.

Better still, this tear fluid works every minute of your waking day. The eye is constantly being bathed by it, in a tiny, steady flow which enters from the tear gland above the upper lid, and leaves through the tear duct to drain into the nose. (This is why you have to blow your nose when you cry.)

The tears are not merely water. They contain, among other antiseptics, a miraculous substance called lysozyme, a germ killer stronger than carbolic acid, yet completely harmless to the eye. This is what helps keep your eyes clear and white.

All day long the blinking lid mops this cleansing fluid over the eye. But during sleep, your eyes are shut and the production of tears is automatically suspended. No tears means no lysozyme, no cleansing and no antiseptic action. Therefore, many patients find their eyes slightly bloodshot and gritty on awakening. When the eyes are open again, the flow of tears starts up once more and, even without bathing or drops, they whiten in 15 to 30 minutes from the action of the lysozyme.

The "bloodshot" eye, which does not clear spontaneously, brings more people to the specialist than any other single symptom. Redness may be slight or severe and may or may not be accompanied by one or more additional complaints such as pain, itching, burning, tearing, sandy sensation, blurring of vision, discharge, pasting of the eyelids or sensitivity to bright light. If these are present, the doctor should be told about them.

The causes of red eye

To list all the causes of congestion of the eye would require a much larger book. The most common causes are:

1. Foreign objects, dusts, fumes, smog, smoke (tobacco or industrial), chemicals, chlorinated pools.

2. Excessive fatigue, sleeplessness, general debility, eyestrain from excessive use under poor conditions, insufficient lighting, insufficient sleep or the need for correct glasses.

3. Allergies, either general allergy or those which specifically affect the eyes such as seasonal plant allergies, allergies to animals or materials, certain cosmetics or dusts.

4. Diseases of nearby structures such as the lids, nose, sinuses, tear ducts, teeth.

5. Infections of the conjunctiva (the thin, transparent membrane which covers the white of the eye and which lines the inside of the lids). Such infections can be acute (sudden and severe) or chronic (stubborn and long drawn out) and most are caused by various germs, such as certain pus-producing bacteria, viruses, fungi, gonorrhea or trachoma.

Some conjunctivitis is contagious. Epidemics of "pink-eye" can spread quickly through a school or a camp if not checked, or better still, prevented. The best prevention is prompt treatment plus isolation. Anyone with a red eye, especially if there is pus or discharge, should use only his own towels and handkerchiefs and keep his hands away from his face. If obliged to touch his face as in using eye drops, the hands should subsequently be scrubbed gently with a soft handbrush, soap and warm water, paying special attention to the folds in the skin, and to the crevices under the fingernails and around the cuticles. Small children, who are likely to forget these precautions, should be kept away from other children in school, camp, swimming pool, or even at home. Parents and teachers must remember that adulthood is no guarantee against contagion and should therefore keep hands away from their own faces — until the eye specialist pronounces the condition no longer contagious.

6. Diseases of the cornea (the transparent, watch-crystal-like window in front of the pupil and iris): injuries, abrasions, embedded foreign particles, ulcers, keratitis (inflammation of the cornea which may be from rheumatic disease, syphilis, vitamin deficiency, infection elsewhere in the body).

7. Glaucoma. The acute type causes much redness and

pain and therefore usually gets attention promptly. The chronic type may develop little or no redness or pain — which makes it more dangerous because it often causes much permanent loss of sight before it is recognized. (See Chapter 2 on glaucoma.)

8. Inflammatory diseases of the structures **within** the eyeball may create some redness. These structures are: the iris, the ciliary body, the choroid, the lens, the vitreous, the retina, the optic nerve. Disease in any of these can be a serious threat to sight. Saving the sight calls for prompt and knowledgeable help not only from the eye specialist but from the family doctor or internist as well — because most diseases inside the eyeball originate elsewhere in the body. The most common of these sources are infection in other organs, rheumatism, diabetes, syphilis, gout, parasites, dental infection, arthritis, etc.

9. Diseases of the structures within the socket behind the eye may cause redness and may be accompanied by swollen eye and lids, bulging eye, impaired vision and sometimes double vision when the eye is prevented from moving properly with the other eye.

Importance of prompt treatment

When the eye is red and inflamed, especially if also blurred and/or painful, the promptness of treatment could make the final outcome sight or blindness. The more delicate an object, the more easily it is damaged, and the harder it is to restore it. This is true of fine watches, fragile china, intricate machines. It is eminently true of the eye. The eye is so delicate that the slightest injury or disease may cause great and permanent harm, whereas a comparable injury elsewhere in the body might scarcely be noticed. For instance, an ulcer on the center of the cornea or a detachment of the retina, persisting and neglected for a few days, could result in permanent impairment of vision.

On the other hand, the very same sensitivity which makes the eye so vulnerable is also one of its best defenses. This sensitivity acts as an early warning system and promptly warns the patient of trouble. The warning signals are: redness, blurring of vision, discomfort in bright light, tearing, pain. It is important to remember that any of these symptoms may not be severe in the beginning, but their early detection and correct treatment at that time can be much more beneficial than any later treatment. Thus, blurring need not be total but may be only slight; sensitiveness to light need not be unbearable; tearing need not be copious; and pain need not be extreme. Any one of these and especially any **combination** of them may spell danger. If they are heeded, an ounce of early treatment is worth a ton of late cure.

See also Chapter 6 on common medical problems in children.

10

The One-Eyed Patient:
One Eye Is Almost As Good As Two

A healthy, two-eyed person hearing the statement "One eye is almost as good as two" rightfully disbelieves it. Obviously, having only one eye cannot be as good as having both. Yet, it is almost as good. Put more correctly, one eye can **do the work** of two, and, more important, continue indefinitely — without wearing out. There are millions of people with but one good eye who go through life quite successfully, doing practically everything two-eyed people do, with a few minor exceptions which I will discuss presently.

In the majority of one-eyed people, the second eye is poor because of amblyopia — from lack of use since early infancy (see Chapter 5 on amblyopia). Never having had binocular vision or true depth perception, they have adapted so well to monocular sight that they may not even know one eye is poor — unless something happens to interfere with the good one.

Those who have started out in life with two normal eyes and later lost the sight of one through disease or injury take a number of months to adjust to their new condition. Their difficulty, at first, is inability to judge distance because of lost binocular vision. They are not safe drivers. They are awkward in sports. They burn their hands at the kitchen range or pour water on the table instead of into a glass. After months, they develop a kind of substitute judgment of depth which enables them to function quite well except in activities requiring true and perfect depth perception, such as landing an airplane, playing outfielder in professional baseball, or performing eye surgery. They usually fail to pass tests for policeman or fireman and cannot get commissions in the armed services.

But for all practical purposes, only the expert can tell that one eye is defective. A moment's reflection will convince anyone that the loss of one leg, or, worse still, one arm, is a far greater hindrance to normal living than the loss of one eye.

Quite another matter is the psychological trauma which follows the actual removal of an eye. Everyone considers the eyes among his most precious possessions. Since he has only two, removal of one can be a shattering experience. Bad as it is, the blow can be softened by proper counselling and presentation of the facts — an important reason for this chapter.

The emotional distress which sets in promptly after the first shock of loss is really anxiety over a series of **NON**-FACTS:

> "My good eye will be overstrained and wear out."
> "I've lost half my sight."
> "I've lost half my field of vision."
> "This is my last chance."
> "I can no longer judge distance."
> "I'll have to quit my job."
> "I'll have to work less (or read less) to preserve my
>   remaining eye."
> "I won't be able to drive."
> "I'll be disfigured."

All of these are simply not true.

I have already pointed out that one eye can carry the

work of two adequately and indefinitely. An eye doesn't wear out. Excessive use may cause fatigue and discomfort which are dispelled by a little rest. In fact, an eye performs better having had **more** work rather than less. One might as well say that a laborer or an athlete wears out his limbs by using them. Obviously, this is not so.

An occasional one-eyed patient finds himself wanting to wear his glasses more than before. He sees better or more comfortably with them, or he feels the remaining eye is better protected from injury by a plastic or shatterproof glass. These reasons are valid and he may wear glasses if he wants to but he is not compelled to do so. And the incidence of injuries to one-eyed patients is no greater than to others. Of course, for any hazardous task it is obviously even more important for him to wear protective glasses (see Chapter 8 on injuries and the prevention of blindness).

"I've lost half my sight and half my field of vision." Not so. While it is indisputable that numerically one eye is half of two eyes, functionally the loss of central vision is zero because he still sees well with the remaining eye. The loss of field (side vision) is only about twenty percent — and he recaptures much of this by constant movement of the eye and head, which he has always done unconsciously even when he used both eyes.

Loss of true depth perception is real. But, as we have already seen, he soon learns to compensate and can function well except where perfection is required. Even so, one of my famous predecessors and teachers, a world-renowned eye surgeon, lost the use of one eye when he was past fifty. He retrained the remaining eye and resumed doing beautiful surgery for years afterward.

If your remaining eye is normal, most states allow you to continue driving.

"Disfigurement." Not so. Even with complete removal of the eye, today's techniques for creating a life-like plastic artificial eye which moves together with the good one make such a condition unrecognizable except on close examination by an expert. All of us who have taught in medical school have played tricks on the senior students by asking them to examine a patient with an artificial eye and getting such diagnoses as syphilis because the pupil didn't dilate, or glaucoma because it felt hard to the touch.

A word of advice to anyone who must have an eye removed: You are not obliged to make the fact public. No one except your family needs to know that you will be wearing an artificial eye — unless you choose to tell them because you would like to receive a lot of sympathy or you wish to talk about your operation.

With all good will, friends may openly engage you in conversations about your artificial eye or you may find them covertly scrutinizing you, trying to discover which one it is. If you are sensitive about such matters, it can be disagreeable.

Therefore, any time it is my unpleasant duty to advise removal of an eye — for a malignant growth or an irreparable and dangerous injury — I always suggest that the patient and the family keep it to themselves. No one else need ever know. It may prevent future embarrassment and may even safeguard a job or a promotion.

11
Window to the Body:
What Your Eyes Reveal
About Your Health

The eye has been called the mirror of the soul. This is debatable. But there is no doubt that it is the window to the body.

It is our great good fortune that the eye is transparent — our only transparent organ. Just as you can look out of it and see the world outside, so I can look into it and discover a great deal about your little world inside.

Looking into the eye (the ophthalmoscope)

Ask any ophthalmologist for his choice of an instrument if he were limited to only one. He would, without hesitation, pick the ophthalmoscope. This instrument permits him to look inside the pupil by sighting along a beam of light which illuminates the inside of the eye. Important structures are revealed: the head of the optic nerve, the arteries and veins of the retina, the macula.

This is what a typical ophthalmoscope looks like:

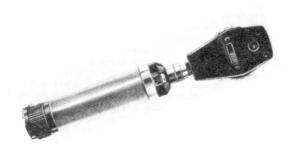

Fig. 7.   An ophthalmoscope.

And this is what we see when we look in:

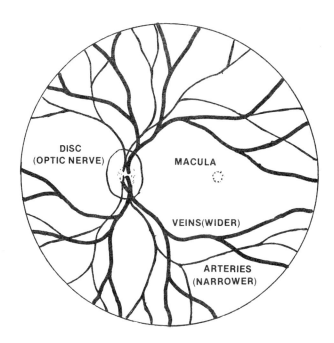

Fig. 8. What the ophthalmologist sees when he uses the ophthalmoscope to look through the pupil at the inside of the eyeball: The disc, just to the left of the center, is the head of the optic nerve. (You also see this in side view on the drawing inside the book cover.) From it, millions of nerve fibers radiate to all parts of the retina. The majority of these fibers go to the macula, the tiny spot to the right of the disc, which is the seat of the sharpest vision (central vision). The nerve fibers are invisible because they are microscopic in size. Seen radiating from the disc are the retinal blood vessels. The wider ones are the branching veins, the narrower ones are the arteries. The veins are blue, the arteries red. The capillaries are too small to be seen except when they become enlarged in certain diseases.

What does the eye reveal?

Abnormalities in the eye often provide the first hint of disease in other parts of the body — sometimes even before the patient himself is aware that there is any trouble. For example, in the course of routine eye examinations, I have discovered unsuspected diabetes in a great many patients who had never had any symptoms.

In other patients, in whom there were baffling symptoms elsewhere in the body, it was the eye examination which revealed the first clue to their cause, as in a recent patient whose persistent headaches had defied many tests and treatments. Here I found an impairment of the peripheral field of vision, so slight that the patient had not noticed it himself. But to me it suggested the possibility of a pituitary gland tumor at the base of the brain. My suspicion was confirmed by a special X-Ray and brain scan. He was cured when the tumor was removed.

This does not mean that such conditions can always be discovered by an eye examination. Obviously, it is not as good as a urine or blood test for diagnosing diabetes; nor does it take the place of neurological tests for locating a brain tumor. But it does show that the eye often provides the first grounds for suspicion and further investigation. Then, other appropriate tests may reveal and locate the disease which might otherwise have been missed. Often the clue leads nowhere. But whether or not it reveals anything, the "window" is there for us to look through.

Space does not permit a detailed description of all the internal conditions disclosed by the eye. A few of the most common and most important are the following:

Diabetes

Diabetes damages the circulation by causing degeneration of the lining and walls of the blood vessels, — first the microscopic capillaries, then the minute arteries and veins. Later, these little vessels become so weakened that they sustain tiny breaks through which bits of blood and serum leak out into the surrounding tissues. These are hemorrhages and they occur most typically in the retina, at the back of the eye. (See below.)

Diabetes may affect the eyes in other ways:

There may be temporary blurring of vision or sudden need for a substantial change in glasses. This is the result of more sugar in the blood and in the ocular fluid, which causes a change in the focus of the eye.

Early cataract may be a sign of diabetes. The same is true of iritis — inflammation of the iris.

More advanced diabetes may cause occasional double vision due to temporary weakness of the muscles which move the eyes.

The most tragic and common of all complications of diabetes is retinal disease. It justifies a more lengthy discussion for two reasons: (1) It is one of the leading causes of blindness; (2) Much of it can be prevented **if** the patient is cooperative.

Diabetic disease of the retina

When I discover this condition in the course of an eye examination, I make it a point to explain its potential seriousness to the patient as clearly and as forthrightly as possible. His understanding is the key to his cooperation. Without this cooperation, no matter how expert the medical advice he receives, he has a good chance of going blind.

But there is a problem here: unfortunately the nature of the condition is such that my explanation cannot be simple or brief. As a result, although he may seem to comprehend while he is in the office, he has forgotten and become confused by the time he has returned home. Sometimes failure to remember is not entirely involuntary, because many diabetics are notorious for ignoring instructions. Such confusion and forgetting are two of the reasons for this book — to provide the patient with something in print to which he may refer at leisure and which he may read and re-read until he understands and, hopefully, obeys.

So, if you are a diabetic or related to one, I urge you to study this chapter carefully because it provides a rare chance for you to practice some real preventive medicine. If you pay attention you may avoid or defer much impairment of sight.

The prevention of blindness from diabetes depends a great deal on the state of your general health, a great deal on how well you manage your diabetes and a little on luck. I mention luck because there will be a few patients who go blind despite the best of care while others will retain good sight despite atrocious neglect. But the lucky ones are few. Don't count on luck when there is so much you **can** do that does make a difference.

Your general health affects your circulation. Anything bad for the circulation is bad for the blood vessels of the eye. What is bad for the circulation? Any chronic illness, obesity, stress, high blood pressure, tobacco, lack of exercise — all take their toll. Age makes matters much worse because with age the arteries become more and more fragile, more brittle, more vulnerable. To all these adversities, add diabetes and you have the seed of much trouble. Now you understand why your doctor keeps warning you about these things especially if you are a senior citizen **and** diabetic.

Measures to preserve your general health may not always be successful, and there is certainly nothing you can do about advancing age, but surely there is hardly any excuse for failure to maintain proper control of the diabetes itself. Your family doctor, internist or specialist in diabetes will carefully and in great detail prescribe and supervise your diet and medication. It is he who periodically evaluates how well your diabetes is controlled. But he cannot go home with you and see that you obey his instructions.

You alone hold the key to success or failure. Your spouse can help. In the office I usually deliver this admonition to **both** halves of a couple and then appoint the other member as the official nag to see that diet and habits are strictly enforced — not six days a week, with a big splurge on Sunday, but seven days, **every** week. I emphasize this because most diabetics are notoriously casual about such matters and it is hard to blame them when they see everyone else having a good time overeating.

Visits to your doctor must be made regularly, at intervals designated by him. The frequency of blood sugar tests should also be determined by him — with one important qualification: you should **not** put yourself on a stricter diet for a few days **before** your blood test. Long ago, I found that some diabetics do this to fool their doctors into thinking they are well controlled because of such a falsely normal blood sugar. In Lawrence we still have a lab technician who makes occasional house calls. If a patient's eyes are doing badly despite a "normal" blood sugar, I sometimes asked the spouse to arrange for an unanticipated blood test on the morning after a forbidden feast. This not only reveals the true blood sugar, but also acts as a warning to the patient when he sees the results of his transgression.

I ask my patients with diabetic disease of the retina to test their own urine each morning — a surprisingly easy and quick procedure. A roll of "test tape" may be purchased at any pharmacy. A small piece of tape is saturated with urine; a change in the color of the tape indicates the presence of any sugar and whether there is a little or a great deal.

This is not a substitute for the blood test but it is

important because it provides **daily** monitoring — a warning at the beginning of each day if you have been doing something wrong. Although it is much cruder than the laboratory test, it does have certain advantages — it can be done at home daily, it requires no puncture of vein or fingertip, it is inexpensive and needs no special skill or training.

What is the outlook for the patient with diabetic disease of the retina? In general, not good. A number of factors make the prognosis even worse: poor control of the diet, high blood sugar, frequent sugar in the urine, poor general health, poor general circulation, long duration of the diabetes, onset of diabetes at an early age, increasing numbers and size of retinal hemorrhages.

In the last few years a new measure of treatment has become available — the laser beam — (see Chapter 14), but this is effective mostly in drying up the small early hemorrhages; it does not prevent new ones, especially if the diabetes continues to remain uncontrolled. Today, we can even restore some sight by operating to remove vitreous clouded by retinal hemorrhage. This also does not prevent new hemorrhages. So your best hope, by far, is still prevention — and the earlier started, the better. There is no one so sad as the patient who had all this explained to him years earlier and, having paid no attention, returns almost blind years later. He cries, "Doctor, help me! I'll do anything you say!" If only he had said that years ago, and abided by it!

On a happier note, I enjoy encouraging my diabetic patients with the following true story: A cousin of mine was a severe diabetic in childhood. By the year insulin was discovered, Betty seemed hopeless and was dying. She was one of the first to be saved by insulin and has remained the picture of health to this day — married, with children, and teaching at a university. She continues the practice of **weighing** her food and calculating her calories, fats, proteins and carbohydrates, — a habit she aquired when young — in addition to taking her daily insulin. Ever since I became an ophthalmologist, I have examined her retina each year and have yet to find a single hemorrhage! Granted, part of this may be luck; but she could never have remained this healthy without her strict observance of the rules.

The brain

The eye is literally part of the brain. In fact, in the embryo, long before the child is born, the brain and the eye are one structure. After birth, they remain intimately connected by way of the optic nerve. Many diseases of the brain — tumor, hemorrhage, abscess, injury, inflammation, syphilis, parasites and impaired circulation — may be revealed by abnormalities found in the course of an eye examination. But a word of caution: it is also possible for any of these diseases to exist **without** producing any eye symptoms. In dealing with the brain, the last word comes from the neurologist, who in turn is aided by sophisticated modern devices like the angiogram, the encephalogram, the brain scan, the sonogram, the tomogram.

Thyroid disease

Certain changes in the eyes may indicate the possibility of thyroid disease. An overactive thyroid may be suspected if the eyes become more prominent or if they appear staring and unusually wide open. Some hyperthyroid patients blink less frequently than normal people. Others have attacks of double vision from disturbances of the eye muscles. Paradoxically, there are instances where these same symptoms appear only **after** the overactivity is cured.

Underactive thyroid may cause puffiness of the eyelids.

For the more definitive diagnosis of thyroid disease your doctor will use various other tests, including chemical analysis of the blood. But often changes in the eye provide the earliest suspicion of the disease.

High blood pressure

This condition is so easily detected during any general medical examination that most patients know about it long before it shows up in the eye. But not all patients see their doctor as regularly as they should. So, there are instances in which, during routine eye examination, I discover evidence of hitherto unsuspected high blood pressure.

This evidence consists of narrowing of the retinal arteries, a change in proportion between the width of the arteries and that of the veins, indentation of the veins by arteries which lie across them, small areas of hemorrhage, swelling, accumulated fluid or atrophy in the retina, or slight swelling of the optic nerve.

In such cases no eye treatment is required, but I send them to their family doctor or internist. Failure to recognize high blood pressure can predispose to serious consequences, including heart disease or stroke. I am often gratified, on later reexamination of the eyes, to see that those ominous findings have disappeared or are much improved with successful reduction of the blood pressure.

Anemia, leukemia, polycythemia

These blood diseases are usually detected by a routine blood count, a common diagnostic procedure. Still, there are patients who have not had a blood test, whose anemia is first suspected because of pallor of the linings of the eyelids (the conjunctiva) or the appearance of a certain kind of small hemorrhage in the retina. Such hemorrhages tend to appear and then absorb after a week or two, so that it is possible for them to be visible at some examinations and not at others.

In polycythemia, a disease in which there are too **many** red blood cells, the retina and its blood vessels may appear a bit dark and congested and there may also be hemorrhages.

Such conditions, when found, require no eye treatment but the patient is sent to his family doctor or internist without delay.

Tobacco

Forgetting, for the moment, its role in the cause of lung cancer and heart disease, the adverse effect of tobacco on the circulation is also well known — so much so that smoking is forbidden in certain circulatory diseases. Anyone who has studied physiology in college remembers how the tiny blood vessels in the web of a frog's foot go into spasm when exposed to a drop of diluted nicotine.

What affects the general circulation affects the circulation in the eye. Use of tobacco to excess sometimes causes tobacco blindness, known technically as tobacco amblyopia, in which the central vision becomes impaired or destroyed with loss of ability to read or discern detail.

In my experience, less extreme effects on the eyes of heavy smokers are sometimes associated with blurring, often combined with numbness or tingling of the fingers — all of which could be attributed to the effect of the tobacco. It is difficult to be certain of a causal relationship here. However, so many of those who could be persuaded to stop or sharply reduce their smoking have reported relief of eye and finger symptoms, that I am compelled to regard it as significant. This has been especially true in older people whose circulation is already affected by age.

Some patients are so heavily addicted that they cannot stop. And if they cannot stop, they are addicts — no matter how unsavory the term. Among these I have had a modest degree of success in reducing the total tobacco intake by convincing them that whatever pleasure or relief they get from the cigarette is from the first puff or two — that they take the remaining eight or ten puffs merely from habit, or to be economical, or merely because it's there. By throwing away three-quarters or more, they waste money but reduce the toxicity by 75 or 80%. Perhaps some of them will even avert lung cancer or a heart attack. It is better still, though, if they break away clean and stop completely. Some of those who merely cut down may go back to full smoking if they are exposed to stress.

Gout

The patient with gout characteristically has much more trouble with his joints than with his eyes, but iritis (inflammation of the iris) is not a rarity in gout. Sometimes he may have the iritis **without** the painful joints, the diagnosis then being made when chemical tests show too much uric acid in the blood.

Local eye treatment of the gouty iritis is usually successful if begun early; the gout itself often responds to drugs and proper diet. If eye treatment is delayed, the iris is sometimes left with some permanent defects and adhesions.

Rheumatic disease and arthritis

These conditions are prevalent but not well understood. Treatment of them is often unsatisfactory. However, patients with such ailments may develop complications in the eyes, usually inflammation of the cornea or the iris. Often the eyes respond to local treatment alone, but it helps if the rheumatic condition can also be alleviated. This necessitates close cooperation between the ophthalmologist and the family doctor.

Syphilis

Syphilis can produce a number of eye diseases, but the most typical are four in number: Severe inflammation of the cornea (keratitis) is seen in small children with inherited syphilis. Iritis may occur in adults with recently acquired syphilis. Inflammation of the interior of the eye, the choroid, retina and optic nerve can be due to the disease later in life. Degeneration and atrophy of the optic nerve and retina occur in the late stages of untreated or inadequately treated syphilis and result in marked impairment of vision.

The appearance of any of the above calls for a simple blood test for syphilis, often still referred to by its old name of Wasserman Test. If the test indicates the presence of the disease, vigorous treatment of both the blood and the eye is often successful in the early stages. The longer it goes untreated, the more the damage and the more difficult the cure.

One source of confusion: Syphilis is known to doctors as "the great imitator." Many diseases appear like syphilis but are not; conversely, many which do not appear so, are. This is why, especially if there is any history of exposure and sometimes even if there is not, doctors, hospitals and clinics include the blood test for syphilis whenever there is occasion for other laboratory tests.

Hardening of the arteries (Arteriosclerosis)

All life consists of six stages — conception, birth, growth, maturity, decline and death. Hardening of the arteries is part of stage five — decline. It begins imperceptibly in youth, rarely becomes noticeable until past middle age and does not present problems until late in life. Although it is as natural and inevitable as death itself, not all people suffer from it to the same extent or in all parts of the body; a few have arteriosclerosis relatively early in life while others show amazingly little evidence of it even in old age. Everyone knows octogenarians who are as bright and alert as they were thirty years earlier.

The circulation of the blood, carried by the arteries and veins to nourish and cleanse the remotest parts of the body, is one of nature's miracles. The blood vessels, beginning with the largest ones near the heart, branch out almost endlessly into smaller and smaller divisions to form millions of microscopic capillaries, each full of moving blood. It is truly astonishing that such a maze of communicating pipes should continue to work without a hitch, without obstruction and without pause, every single minute, hour, day and year for many decades.

All parts of the body are dependent on the circulation of the blood. Some organs, such as the heart, brain, or eye — because they are highly specialized and delicate — are more easily disabled by defects in the circulation. The amount of disability depends on how much arteriosclerosis exists and which part of the eye is involved. It may be slight and develop slowly like the small reduction in sharpness of sight which comes on gradually with age. It may cause symptoms which are annoying but not serious, like itching of the lids or spots and flashes — all of which may be from minor disturbances in circulation.

But the more severe circulatory diseases of the eye can be very distressing. Great reduction in vision may be the result of advanced degrees of sclerosis of all the arteries of the retina. This is not a common condition except in the very old or very senile who usually are already greatly handicapped by general arteriosclerosis in other parts of the body.

A more common disease is degeneration, not of the entire retina, but only of its center. It is called macular degeneration.

Macular degeneration

You will recall that the retina is capable of two kinds of vision: central and peripheral, each important in its own way. With **central** vision we distinguish **detail**, both at close range as in reading and sewing, and at a distance, as with traffic lights and road signs. **Peripheral** vision gives us the perception of our **surrounding** environment, the vision which makes us aware of objects and movement not in the direct line of sight but to the sides. Peripheral vision prevents us from colliding with other people or cars when we walk or drive; it is used in those tasks not requiring discernment of detail.

Central vision is performed by the macula, a tiny spot in the very center of each retina. Peripheral vision is performed by all the rest of the retina, at least 99% of it, outside the macula.

In macular degeneration it is this minute area at the center which deteriorates, gradually blurring and eliminating **central** vision but leaving most of the peripheral vision intact. This deterioration may be a senile, arteriosclerotic process but it sometimes occurs prior to old age, from hereditary or other causes not yet clearly understood.

If the macular degeneration is limited to only one eye, patients continue to function normally. In fact, many of them are not aware of the condition unless they happen to close the good eye. This is difficult to believe, but it is a common occurrence in every ophthalmologist's office — a patient with dense, obviously old scarring of one macula, yet not aware that he is using only one eye!

Where the condition occurs in both eyes or, having taken place earlier in one eye and now developing in the second eye, it is noticed promptly. Now we have an otherwise healthy person who would have functioned quite normally for his age but cannot because of reduced or absent central vision. If such an individual happens to be already retired, it means at worst a reorientation of goals, hobbies and diversions. If he is still working, unless the work requires no sharp central vision, as perhaps in some types of manual labor, he may have to give up his job or be retrained for some other kind of occupation, a task not always easy for an older person.

Treatment of macular degeneration is not rewarding, especially when it is due to deterioration of the circulation alone. Some degenerations are not entirely circulatory but look and act like them, and only an ophthalmologist, with the help of a special device called an angiogram, can distinguish this type and, perhaps, arrest the process with application of a finely focused laser beam (see Chapter 14). This treatment is entirely without discomfort to the patient, often requires no hospitalization and usually not even an anesthetic because he feels nothing at all. However, it is a (relatively) new method which demands specialized training and skill and the use of very delicate and highly sophisticated equipment, is not entirely free of risk to adjacent areas, and therefore is not undertaken lightly, without weighing these risks against the possible benefits.

Early or lesser degrees of macular degeneration may be aided by optical devices known as low-vision aids. These are various types of magnifying lenses, spectacles, telescopic or microscopic devices and even projectors which throw enlarged images onto a screen or television receiver. They can be cumbersome, expensive and limited in their use but in some instances a tremendous boon, even making the difference between idleness and employment. Often, they are a disappointment or can become so if the degeneration continues to progress. They do have one advantage — it is usually possible to try them before going to the expense of purchasing one.

It is most important that every patient with macular degeneration be made aware of one fact: he is **not** going blind. When he finds his central vision failing, his first fear is that he will soon be helpless. This is not so. He may be unable to read, sew or work at fine tasks, but the **peripheral** vision in such patients is practically never impaired. He will always be able to get about unaided and, with some limitation, attend to himself, his household, his meals, recreation and shopping.

What can be done for arteriosclerosis?

At present very little. Although much research is in progress, little that is definite has been discovered so far. Our ideas of cause and relief are based more on experience and common sense than on hard scientific fact. Apart from age and heredity, some of the culprits we suspect are faulty diet, overweight, stress, tobacco, lack of exercise and chronic debility. Prevention or treatment would aim to eliminate as many of these as possible.

For temporary improvement, the internist or the ophthalmologist sometimes prescribes various medications which seem to help the patient by improving his circulation. I have also found that in older patients small doses of brandy or any hard liquor (2 or 3 teaspoons) taken 4 times daily before meals and at bedtime give them a sense of well-being and better vision. It is quite possible that some day our approach will be more scientific and the outlook more encouraging.

More about spots, floaters and flashes

Minor disturbances of circulation in patients over forty-five may cause spots, floaters or even flashes. Usually they are harmless, though annoying and, at first, frightening. Spots or threads are translucent and without well-defined shape. They appear to 'float' in the air before the eyes and move with the eyes, rarely in the direct line of sight but usually a bit away from the center. If they do happen to persist in the direct line of sight, they can interfere somewhat with reading of print or music. Some patients report that they disappear for periods of time, then reappear. They practically never cause any significant impairment in vision.

Those spots that are due to circulatory disturbance are likely to be more prominent under circumstances adverse to the circulation, such as stress, anxiety, fatigue, illness or heavy smoking. They may diminish or disappear when, on proper advice or medication, these adverse circumstances are corrected.

Other spots are the result of minor changes within the vitreous itself. With age, the vitreous body which has been a jelly-like liquid tends to become thinner and more fluid. In the process it shrinks a bit and draws forward, then separates from the retina. This is sometimes referred to as "detachment of the vitreous," but in no sense is it anything like detachment of the retina. It is quite harmless. When the vitreous changes in this fashion, some portions of it condense and are seen by both the patient and the doctor as translucent threads or spots. They need no treatment, and most patients, after being reassured that they are in no danger, become adjusted to their presence.

Flashes, with or without the presence of spots, are an indication of irritation of the retina. When other body structures are stimulated, there is transmitted to the brain a sensation of touch or pain or heat or cold. The retina is capable of transmitting only one sensation — light, just as the nerves of the ear and nose can transmit only sound or smell. If one were able to touch the retina with a sharp pin, the brain would get a message not of a pinprick but of a flash. Thus, when the contracting vitreous exerts a tiny pull on the retina, or when a minute blood vessel in the retina responds to stress or momentary rise in blood pressure, the patient may experience the only kind of sensation that the nerve from the retina knows how to transmit — a flash.

While flashes are often harmless, they are sometimes a danger signal, an early warning of retinal detachment (see Chapter 4). Persons with persistent spots or flashes should be examined by an ophthalmologist because only he can determine whether they are harmless or not.

12
The Mind and the Eye

Our familiar word "psychosomatic" is made up of "psyche" (mind) and "soma" (body) — any part of the body including the eye. The term usually defines an illness or the symptom of an illness whose cause is mental or emotional rather than physical or organic. The simplest example of the distinction between the two is the act of weeping. When caused by grief it is "crying" (psychosomatic), when caused by a foreign object or by a head cold it is "tearing" (physical).

An important feature of the psychosomatic ailment is that its nature or even its very existence can be difficult to prove. Organic disease can usually be detected with fair precision by the doctor's own senses or specific laboratory tests which yield a definite answer to the question : Is disease absent or present? For example, given a patient who has just developed blurred vision: if the cause is physical I can **see** the cloudy cornea or the cataract or the retinal detachment; I can **feel** the hardened eye of glaucoma and even measure it with a tonometer; I can **hear** with my stethoscope applied to the closed eye the sound of the exaggerated pulse made by the tumor in the socket behind the eyeball; I can **measure** the eye, and if it is astigmatic, correct the blur with proper glasses; if I **discover** a defect in the field of vision I may suspect a brain tumor or tobacco poisoning; the laboratory test **tells** me the patient has syphilis or diabetes; the X-Ray **shows** me a bone tumor pressing on the optic nerve.

All these are definite. I **know** they are there because I

can see, hear or feel them. I can **prove** they are there and any other doctor with the same training and experience can do the same. Medically, we call such findings **objective**.

Subjective findings — so called because only the **subject** (the patient) is aware of them — are the prominent feature of psychosomatic ailments. Here, although the **result** is sometimes tangible (an attack of asthma, palpitation or even glaucoma), the **cause** is usually mental or emotional, and often examination discloses no physical disease. However, I must do such an examination, including all necessary tests, to rule out organic disease before I can conclude that the problem is mental in origin. And even when I have come to this conclusion, I cannot always be certain. Many things are still unknown. And many ailments are so slight or so early that they are simply undetectable until further advanced or more obvious.

Even if all the tests are negative, it does not imply that a psychosomatic ailment cannot be real, that the patient is not suffering, or that he is a malingerer. Pain is always real as are other symptoms, even though their **cause** may be mental or emotional. Emotions can produce real illness. A famous case, fortunately rare, was that of a woman with asthma, a disease whose cause is not always apparent. Her attacks were severe enough to threaten her life. In desperation, she went to Arizona where she felt fine. On her return to the East, the attacks recurred. Her husband then sold his business and they both moved to Arizona, but her attacks worsened. In short, she was allergic to her husband. Since their divorce, they are both well and happy and live in the East.

Sometimes emotions cause a baffling mixture of psychosomatic illness combined with real disease, as with the mother who managed to keep her son from marrying by having a "heart attack" which succeeded in driving away any girl he brought home. Examinations and electrocardiograms always proved normal. When the son finally realized that the mother's condition was psychosomatic, he found still another girl and married her. At the wedding the mother had a real heart attack and died. (Thereby launching her son on a psychosomatic career of his own.)

I have always warned my students that a patient with a psychosomatic ailment is as much subject to serious physical disease as anyone else; that a patient who has long suffered from headaches from tension or depression can **also** subsequently develop pain in the head from glaucoma.

Sometimes what is one person's psychosomatic illness can be another's organic disease:

Years ago there was a popular motion picture, "Dark Victory," in which Bette Davis suffers from visual disturbance cause by a brain tumor. For the following few years, I was consulted by hundreds of patients with visual disturbances who thought they had brain tumors. All but two, after careful examination, turned out to be perfectly normal. The two who did indeed have brain tumors were thus discovered early and cured by prompt surgery, thanks to Bette Davis. Had it not been for her, these two might have gone undiscovered until too late.

An example nearer home, involving the eyes, is that of a person with glaucoma. Glaucoma is not psychic in origin, but when present it can be worsened by stress:

A sensitive and apprehensive patient of forty happened to have her first attack of glaucoma while I was out of town, necessitating treatment by a colleague in my absence. Subsequently, the pressure in her eyes was well controlled by her use of drops. But whenever she heard I was out of town or planning to leave, she would suffer another glaucoma attack. The glaucoma was real, and with each attack the pressure measured alarmingly high. But triggering each attack was a purely psychic insecurity and apprehension. It became so troublesome that my staff had to take elaborate precautions to prevent her from discovering my absence. Her attacks finally stopped only after I operated on both her eyes, creating tiny safety valves which automatically reduced the eye pressure whenever it rose.

Too often we forget that children may also have psychosomatic symptoms, and that, in their own little sphere, problems in proportion to their size might be very real:

Jimmy, aged five, was brought to me because he had recently begun blinking violently. The more his parents puzzled over it and questioned him, the more he blinked. Careful examination revealed no physical cause or other obvious reason. They denied any emotional stress. My next question: "Are there any other children?" "Yes, a baby sister, eight weeks old." When I ventured that this might be an emotional reason for the blinking, the mother vehemently rejected the idea, explaining that the boy loved his new sister. The following dialogue then took place:

> Dr. E. "How long are you married?"
> Mrs. G. "Seven years."
> Dr. E. "Happily?"
> Mrs. G. "Yes."
> Dr. E. "For seven years you've had the undivided affection of your husband all to yourself. Suppose this evening he walked in with a second wife, do you think you might start blinking?"

Enough said. The mother was convinced that the blinking was psychosomatic. At my suggestion, the parents began lavishing as much attention on the boy as they had on the newborn. The child's blinking stopped several weeks later.

CAUTION: Stories such as the one about blinking do not always have a happy ending. I remember a two-year-old whose blinking had been diagnosed by the parents as psychosomatic. A month elapsed before they brought her to me and I found an ulcer on the center of one cornea. By then, it had caused enough severe scarring over the pupil to impair the vision permanently.

This is why a doctor makes sure, by careful examination, that there is no **organic** disease before he makes a diagnosis of a psychosomatic condition — especially in small children who cannot express their complaints in words.

Psychosomatic problems are part of every physician's practice, no matter what his specialty. All medicine is detective work. One of its great attractions is the constant battle of wits — the doctor's training, experience and alert reasoning pitted against the mystery of human affliction — physical or mental. The culprit could be obvious and apprehended promptly — like the murderer standing over the corpse with a smoking gun, or the rusty piece of steel imbedded in the cornea, causing a painful ulcer. Or the culprit could be well hidden and elusive like the spy who is caught only after five hundred pages of the novel, or the obscure disease discovered only after long, drawn-out and painstaking investigation.

In some instances, just as in police work, the solution is never found.

Psychosomatic symptoms or diseases can mimic most physical ailments. They are so numerous that in a busy practice we are likely to see at least one every day, and to describe them all would be impossible. In fact I might be doing the susceptible reader a disservice, creating ailments by suggestion, if I haven't done so already.

What can be done?

Now, assuming that we have gone through a careful examination, including all necessary tests and consultations, have ruled out organic disease as well as is humanly possible and are convinced that we are dealing with a psychosomatic condition. What can be done about it?

Sometimes the procedure is simple. I try to find out by merely asking, "Are you aware of anything that's upsetting you?" A direct response can prove to be the solution. A patient, frightened because a friend had a serious illness, followed by blindness or death, has already been reassured by my finding no disease. She is cured when made aware of the causal relationship between blurred vision and the friend's tragedy.

Sometimes the solution cures the symptom only to have it crop up elsewhere. A boy with serious problems at school but who thought he needed glasses was cured of twitching eyelids when reassured that no glasses were necessary. A few weeks later he developed a twitch of his neck muscles.

Sometimes nothing needs to be done. As in organic illness, the patient gets better by himself — in spite of the doctor rather than because of him.

Sometimes there is no solution. A young mother saw flashes and spots. Careful examination disclosed no detachment of the retina. Questioning revealed that her husband had recently deserted her and three small children. She readily understood the connection with her symptoms. What I didn't tell her was that she was lucky, under the circumstances, to get away with mere flashes and not a stomach ulcer.

Often the answer is not so readily forthcoming. The patient may not know or be unwilling to tell. The situation may be too complicated and call for more facts or consultation with someone more knowledgeable. Our most precious resource here is the family doctor who knows much more than the specialist about the patient, about his family, environment and problems.

The family practitioner has become more rather than less important in modern medicine. Society has begun to recognize this. The main reason for specialization is quite simply the staggering increase in medical knowledge — much more in the last fifty years than in the previous five thousand! Because no one doctor can possibly cope with all this information, the practice of medicine has become fragmented. It has been aptly said that the specialist is one who knows more and more about less and less. Precisely because of this, the family doctor is important. With his general knowledge of the entire field, he pulls all the loose ends together into a picture of the patient as a person, a whole individual, rather than an eye or a kidney or a joint.

Sometimes the cause is so obscure and deep-seated that we cannot identify the intolerable emotional disturbance which the patient has converted into a more tangible, more tolerable eye ailment. In such cases, either the family doctor or I recommend consultation with a psychiatrist, often with gratifying and prompt improvement.

Foolishly, some patients still think there is some stigma attached to consulting a psychiatrist. I point out that psychiatrists are merely another kind of medical specialist and that innumerable average and ordinary people with emotional problems go to them and are helped.

Nor need anyone feel that there is a stigma attached to having emotional or psychosomatic problems. It is only the proverbial contented cow which is not, at one time or other, subject to stress. In humans, with a brain so marvelously complex and organized that it has the potential to explore the innermost atom or outermost space, to compose a symphony or write a love letter, the miracle is that there is not **more** psychosomatic disturbance. Not all people react alike. As with physical disease, some of us have more resistance than others. But it is rare that a serious psychic problem leaves us unaffected, whether we know it or not.

As for the doctor, he is fully aware that in psychosomatic disease the problems can be very real. Cure may be difficult or impossible; he may have to call for help. But it is in this sphere that he meets his greatest challenge — a challenge which requires training, experience, insight, judgment, concern and patience.

13
Contact Lenses

Doctor, can I wear contact lenses?

Yes, if you really need them. Over the last ten years, contact lenses have been so improved that almost anyone can wear them. Now the question is no longer "Can I wear them?" but "Should I?" In other words, since modern design has eliminated most technical obstacles, is it now desirable to wear them instead of spectacles?

Today over ten million Americans wear contact lenses; over a million new ones each year.

What do you mean, "If I really need them?"

Not all people should get contact lenses just because they think they need them or simply because they are "something new."

Contact lenses are a little more trouble to put on and remove than ordinary spectacles. This makes them impractical for persons who wear glasses only occasionally, or only for special tasks such as reading or driving. Such people would be silly to bother with contact lenses. This is also true if you wear glasses without really needing them. (See Chapter 1, "Doctor, Do I Need Glasses?")

What are the reasons for wearing contact lenses?

There are four main reasons. They are: appearance, better vision, safety, or irregular cornea.

Appearance

The vast majority of those who wear contact lenses do so because they cannot go without glasses and prefer contacts purely for the sake of appearance.

Because most men are not quite as concerned as women about how they look, there are many more female contact lens wearers than male. No one need be apologetic about this; we should all have the privilege of appearing as we please.

Fortunately, wearing glasses no longer carries quite the social stigma it did years ago when Ogden Nash wrote, with fair accuracy for those days, "Men don't make passes at girls who wear glasses." And I still remember the shrieks of derision that greeted me the morning I entered my fourth grade classroom wearing glasses, and how I discovered, when they called me "four-eyes" and kept me off the ball team, that I didn't really need them — then or since.

Today the picture is different. Since the introduction of high style in eyeglasses, since the name of the frame may be that of a famous designer (at quadruple the cost), since every young lady and her mother must have several pairs to go with different costumes, — those who used to want contact lenses because others wore them, now are content to wear stylish oversized spectacles instead.

Yet there are many who prefer contact lenses because they still do not wish to be seen wearing glasses. This is especially true for those who must wear very thick glasses — the very near-sighted, the very far-sighted, the very astigmatic or those who have had cataract surgery. (See Chapter 3 on cataract.)

Better vision

The contact lens has still another advantage: better and more natural vision. When you wear a heavy glass, it focuses perfectly in the center, but not toward the edge. The thicker it is, the worse the side vision. This is not true of the contact because (1) it is close to the eye, (2) it is very thin and (3) it moves with the eye. The center of the contact lens always remains lined up with the pupil, producing good peripheral (side) vision in every direction — a great advantage over the thick glass when it comes to sports, motoring, hunting and combat. Also, contact lenses do not become foggy in cold weather.

Safety

In sports, the contact lens wearer finds another benefit: safety. In the past, many young people avoided sports because of their glasses. Now they may participate in comfort and safety. The exception to this is swimming — not that contacts are not safe, but because they may float away and be lost.

Irregular cornea (keratoconus)

The normal cornea is perfectly curved and helps the eye to focus perfectly. A rare kind of deformity distorts this curvature, so that the surface of the cornea, instead of being round, becomes cone-shaped and irregular. This is called conical cornea, or keratoconus (see p. 251).

Before the days of contact lenses, people with keratoconus suffered from poor vision which became gradually and increasingly so distorted that even with glasses they could perform only the crudest tasks. Worse still, this ailment often struck young adults who found their jobs or their careers interrupted at a critical time in their lives.

Today these peoples' lives are completely changed. Miraculously, a contact lens restores good vision. Now a faulty, irregular corneal surface which distorted the image can be "paved over" with a perfectly curved contact lens. This artificial, new corneal surface, now normally focused, allows the image passing into the eye to remain sharp and clear.

What are the reasons for not wearing contacts?

Nuisance, cost, risk, and intolerance.

Nuisance

Contacts are more trouble than glasses to clean, to put on and take off. But nuisance is a relative term. If you are quite comfortable with spectacles and you wear them only occasionally and only for special purposes, you would consider contacts a nuisance and should not get them.

On the other hand, if you wear heavy glasses constantly, you might find the task of inserting and removing contacts worth the trouble.

Cost

Cost is a definite consideration. Hard contacts can cost many times as much as glasses; and soft lenses are about twice as expensive as hard ones. Because contacts are lost more easily than glasses, the cost of replacement can become substantial.

Risk

See below under "Are contacts safe?" and "What are the dangers?"

Intolerance

See below under "Do some people accept contacts more readily than others?"

What exactly is a contact lens?

A contact lens is a tiny paper-thin, almost weightless plastic lens which is worn on the front surface of the eye. It is so called because it stays in "contact" with the cornea and moves with the movement of the eyeball.

How does it stay on the eye?

To understand how the lens stays on the cornea without falling off, take a clean flat piece of glass, moisten it and place it against a clean window pane. It clings to the pane, yet slides about easily as long as there is a bit of moisture between the two surfaces. The contact lens does the same except that instead of being flat like the window, it is curved exactly like your cornea. If the curvature is not correctly suited to your particular cornea, it will not stay on properly or may be uncomfortable. Corneal curvatures are not the same in all patients; therefore the doctor carefully measures the surface of your cornea with a special instrument called a keratometer to make sure that the lens you get is a perfect fit for that particular surface.

Then, while this lens is being made, the proper prescription to correct near-sightedness or far-sightedness is incorporated into it. You thus wear on your cornea practically the same prescription you have been wearing in your spectacles.

What is the difference between 'hard' and 'soft' lenses?

Both are made of plastic materials and work on the same principle which I just explained, but each has certain advantages and disadvantages.

The hard or conventional contact lenses have been available longer, have been subject to more improvements, are less fragile, last longer, are easier to handle, easier to store, easier to clean, do not need special methods and apparatus for sterilizing, do not soak up medication, and cost about half as much as the soft lenses.

Soft lenses are usually more easily tolerated by the relatively few patients who cannot wear the hard ones. Because they absorb the warm tear fluid they are not only more pliant but feel more natural in the eye. Their softness makes them less likely to scratch the eye if inserted carelessly. But while they absorb tear fluid they can also absorb bacteria and fungi which are dangerous to the eye. Therefore they must be sterilized every day — by boiling or by soaking in special solutions. Also, being more fragile, they are more easily torn while handling; and they need to be replaced much sooner than hard lenses.

Are there other kinds of contact lenses?

There are, under investigation, new types of contact lenses designed for long-term wear — weeks, months, perhaps years. Present contacts must be removed daily because they do not breathe — that is, they do not allow quite enough oxygen, carbon dioxide or heat to pass to and from the cornea. Hopefully, within the next two or three years, lenses of new materials which correct this drawback will become available. When this happens your ophthalmologist will certainly know about it.

Also, both hard and soft lenses are constantly being modified and improved, and semi-soft lenses are under investigation. They combine some of the advantages and drawbacks of both the hard and the soft lenses.

There are also larger lenses which rest on the sclera, or white of the eye, allowing the central or corneal part to lie in front of the cornea without touching it.

Are contact lenses safe?

Yes, reasonably safe. If you bear in mind that nothing is completely free of hazard, I would call them safe. Millions of people wear them and mishaps are very rare. As for the ingredients that go into the lenses, the U.S. Food and Drug Administration makes as certain as it can that they are harmless before allowing their use.

What are the dangers of contact lenses?

The great majority of problems are created by the wearer, rather than the lens.

Lack of cleanliness is the most important. Lens wearers should always remember to wash their hands before touching their contact lenses. The tiniest bit of dirt picked up from your fingers can not only be painfully irritating to your eye, but can also scratch and damage the contact lens.

Cleaning the lens is equally vital. The doctor who prescribes them will give you instructions; they should be followed to the letter, especially with the soft lenses.

Rough handling during insertion or removal can be a real hazard (a little less with the soft lenses). Carelessness could cause an abrasion of the cornea — a painful mishap which disables the wearer for days or weeks (see pp. 127-8).

Overwearing can cause trouble. New wearers are instructed how long they may wear their contacts and how to increase their wearing time. Even after they are fully acclimated, I advise most patients to remove them after eight to twelve hours. Those who can and wish to wear them sixteen hours a day are urged to remove them for half an hour in the late afternoon and then to reinsert them. Frankly, many do not bother to do this and seem to suffer no harm, wearing them all day every day for many years.

In no case should contacts be worn during sleep unless specifically permitted by the doctor. If the eye is red or inflamed (see Chapter 9) the contact is generally omitted.

If a foreign object gets into the eye, the contact should

be removed promptly and placed in its carrying case which you should always have with you. The lens lying loose in pocket or purse becomes soiled and may be lost or damaged.

Irregularity or roughness of the lens itself can be dangerous, especially in the hard lens. It can be caused by a chipped or cracked edge. Fortunately this is extremely rare, considering the fragility of this tiny object. The best way to avoid it is by careful handling and by a moment's inspection each day before wearing.

If a defective lens is inserted, you are very likely to sense it immediately; any new or unaccustomed irritation or scratchiness calls for prompt removal and inspection. If you find nothing to explain it, the supplier or the doctor should check the lens and the eye before you resume wearing it. Since this hardly ever happens to both lenses at once, there is no objection to using the one comfortable lens (or no lenses, just spectacles) for a day or so until the suspicious lens can be checked.

What is the best way to insert and to remove contact lenses?

The procedure is so simple that millions of people do it effortlessly once they have learned. However, it is not advisable for the new wearer to learn from a book; a demonstration is so much better, quicker, and safer. You are entitled to this instruction as part of the fitting process. For most people, one or two sessions are enough. But before you go home with your new contacts, make sure you have understood how to handle them. Do not hesitate to ask questions. Practice inserting and removing them in the presence of the doctor or his aide — until you have confidence in what you are doing — before you leave.

If you have difficulty with the contacts the first few times, postpone wearing them until you have returned to the office for more instruction.

What if I cannot remove the contact lenses when I am at home?

You have no choice but to return to the office to have them removed and to receive more instruction. However, this happens very rarely because removing them is even easier than putting them on.

What do I do if I put on a contact lens and find that I do not see any better?

This can happen for one of several reasons. You may not have placed it on the cornea; it may have been lost during insertion; or it may have slipped up or down under either lid or into either corner of the eye. You may have used the wrong lens or the wrong solution.

To avoid loss, it is best at first to work over a clean, white, undecorated towel, so that the lens is easily found if it falls on it.

A misplaced lens in the eye can usually be seen in a mirror (a magnifying mirror if you are far-sighted), then removed and re-inserted correctly. Some dextrous persons can coax the lens back on to the cornea by a combination of rolling the eye and gentle manipulation of the eyelids. There is some risk here of irritating the cornea if you are not light-handed, or if you keep trying too long or too hard.

Is it possible to put on someone else's contacts by mistake?

Yes, especially if others in the family wear them. This can be avoided by always putting contacts, directly after removal, into their own carrying case. Make sure the case has your name on it.

Is it possible to interchange the right and left lenses by mistake?

Yes, if on removing them from your eyes, you fail to put

each lens in its proper compartment, labeled R and L. As an additional precaution, I recommend the right lens of each pair be marked, when it is made, with a tiny black dot near its edge.

Is the kind of wetting solution important?

Yes. Use only the solution recommended when you get your lenses. Make sure you look at the label on the bottle **each** time you use it so that you do not make a mistake and use the wrong solution or some other fluid not even meant for the eye.

At what age may contacts be worn?

Contacts may be worn at any age, even by very small infants after removal of congenital cataracts as well as by eighty or ninety year olds after removal of senile cataracts.

Is my fourteen year old daughter too young for contact lenses?

No, but if possible, it would be a little better to wait until she is older. I have prescribed contacts for many children, even under fourteen, but only when they and their parents have insisted, and then only after I had carefully enumerated the drawbacks.

What are the drawbacks in the young child?

The younger the child, the less dependable she is about care, cleanliness, overwearing, removal at bedtime; and the more often lenses are lost, mislaid, or roughly used — especially if they had been handed the child as a ready gift. Children who have had to get a job and earn the considerable cost of contacts hardly ever lose them.

Also, the younger the child the more sensitive the eyes and the more difficulty in becoming accustomed to the lenses. No matter how well fitted, a contact lens is a foreign object and feels a little scratchy at first. A young child who fails to accept it and thus becomes conditioned against it may have greater difficulty later on than an older child who is better able to tolerate the initial small discomfort.

I want my daughter to wear contacts to improve her appearance, but she is reluctant. Should I urge her?

Lack of motivation is the greatest obstacle to the wearer's tolerance of the lens. I flatly refuse to prescribe contact lenses for a child when it is the parent who wants them for social reasons and the child is reluctant. Such attempts always fail.

On the other hand, the child who wants them badly, perhaps for good reason — such as thick glasses, very poor vision without glasses, or ridicule by her peers — will have no difficulty at practically any age. The best candidate is such a child who finally gets contacts despite moderate resistance from her parents and from me, who has been put off by me for six months or a year, thereby further increasing her motivation, and who has had to get a job to pay for them.

Do some people accept contact lenses more readily than others?

Yes. Ocular sensitivity varies enormously even among adults. It is almost always greater in children and less in most older persons. A good example of this is the difference in tolerance to mild eye drops. Some patients will hardly blink, others will grimace and squeeze the lids, rub the eyes, or even jump up out of the chair. I often use the reaction to an eye drop as a test of whether the patient will tolerate contacts readily. In fact, to accustom the eyes to the sensation prior to fitting contact lenses, I sometimes ask the patient to use drops at home a few times daily for a few weeks.

I now wear bifocals constantly. Can I get bifocal contact lenses?

There are such things as bifocal contact lenses, but few people have been happy with them.

There are several possible alternatives, none as convenient as bifocal spectacles. You could wear contacts focused only for distance, and put on reading glasses in addition (over them) whenever you look at anything close. Or, you could wear contacts focused only for near, and put on distance glasses over them for driving, theater, television — or whenever you need to see sharply in the distance.

More often, in such situations, if the patient does not require constant sharp focus, both distant and close, I prescribe contacts focused for about twenty inches (about one and one half times as far as ideal reading distance). These will suffice for most tasks performed at middle distance. Some people wear such a contact lens only at work, focused appropriately for their working distance. On the rare occasions when such a person needs sharp distant vision or fine near vision, she puts on a pair of glasses (while still wearing the contacts) with appropriate additional focusing power for either distance or fine print.

The simplest solution — if you are not helpless without your bifocals — is not to bother with contact lenses at all. Just take off your bifocals when appearance is important, and wear them only when you need sharp vision, far or near. You may be uncomfortable or your vision blurred, but you will do yourself no harm whatever. Read the chapter "Doctor, Do I Need Glasses?" and you will understand.

Can contacts be colored so that my eyes look blue?

Yes, they can be made in any color. Blue is the most popular.

Can contacts be replaced if I lose them or break them?

Yes, easily, but it may take a few days or longer.

Can I get insurance against lost or broken contacts?

Yes, most people do, at the time they get their lenses. The cost is nominal compared to that of the lenses. It is higher for the soft lenses — but more necessary because of the higher cost of replacement. Insurance usually covers most, but not all the cost of replacement. This subjects you to a small penalty every time the insurance company replaces your lost contacts.

Should I have a spare pair of contacts?

Only if the cost is no object or if you are so dependent upon the contacts that you cannot work or study for the week or so that you wait for a replacement. Even so, most people can get along wearing their spectacles or one contact lens temporarily.

I have heard of using special contact lenses as a means of reducing near-sightedness or eliminating it entirely. Is this possible?

This is a matter of some controversy. The procedure, known as orthokeratology — using contacts to increasingly "mold" the cornea — is considered by some ophthalmologists a bit risky, with the chance of ultimate damage to the cornea from pressure and interference with its nutrition. Also it is a bit expensive, involving not one pair of contacts but a number of changes over a period of two or more years.

It is true that some people experience a modest reduction in myopia after wearing their contact lenses a few weeks. In my experience, this is usually not permanent and the near-sightedness returns to its original condition when the contacts are left off. The reduction, if it occurs, is rarely sufficient to allow the patient to discard glasses or contacts entirely.

Much research and proof will be required before the procedure is considered effective and harmless. In the meantime we try to keep an open mind on the subject.

Does the wearing of contact lenses prevent near-sightedness from getting worse?

In most cases, probably no. The reason some wearers think so is a bit complicated: Myopia usually increases fastest during children's growing years, then levels off or stops when they reach full height. It is at this time, in the late teens, that most young people begin to wear contact lenses. They mistakenly give credit to the contact lenses for stopping the increase of their myopia — something which would have happened anyway, with or without contact lenses.

Would you yourself wear contact lenses?

Patients sometimes ask me this. I wouldn't be bothered. But then, I don't have to be beautiful. If I needed glasses I would wear spectacles, and then only when I wanted to see better. In my family, my wife long ago learned to wear her glasses for distance only, so she does not need to bother with contact lenses. Of my children, only one wears contacts most of the time, another rarely, the rest not at all.

14
Recent Discoveries
in Ophthalmology

Along with the rockets and satellites of the space age have come quieter but equally spectacular developments in medical science, which enable us to do much more for you than we could a few short years ago. Today we can diagnose much more accurately and cure more easily than ever before, thanks to the efforts and talents of a large number of research workers.

These are very special people. They are prodded by insatiable curiosity and fueled by inexhaustible energy. Their reward is the excitement of their search, the solution of their problems, the application of these solutions to the general welfare, and, occasionally, the recognition of their achievement by the public and the profession. Most of them receive very little economic gain from their efforts, but publish their findings for the free use of society and of other investigators.

All research is a gamble, the playing of an educated hunch. For every Edison or Pasteur there are thousands who remain unknown; for every Nobel prize winner there are thousands who are barely recognized, but who go on increasing our knowledge, diminishing our pain, improving our vision and prolonging our lives. To them, we doctors and our patients will always be in tremendous debt.

While we are on the subject of research, the matter of its financing is of intimate concern to everyone who might some day become sick — meaning all of us. Research costs money, lots of it. Less money means less research, which in turn spells more suffering and more blindness.

Research funds come from two sources: private donors and government grants.

In the private sector, much of the funding has been engineered by an organization called Research to Prevent Blindness. Started years ago by Dr. Jules Stein, an ophthalmologist turned businessman, and financed largely by him, this organization has funneled millions of dollars into the support of research projects which have enormously improved life, sight and health everywhere. A number of other non-profit organizations such as "Fight for Sight" and Lions Clubs have done excellent work financing research and various forms of eye care. All of them greatly deserve the generous support of everyone who appreciates the importance of vision.

The principal source of research money is the federal government. Much of what you will read about in this chapter is, in one way or another, an outgrowth of the tremendous explosion of scientific knowledge during the post-sputnik era. It was then that our government was most generous in its support of scientific research. It was then that the subsidized labor of only a few thousand scientists made America the undisputed world leader in scientific and medical progress, revealing one more reason for the greatness and intrinsic altruism which, despite its acknowledged imperfections, characterizes our country. It was then that the discoveries were made which led to our high percentage of recent Nobel prize winners.

Unfortunately, recent ill-advised cuts in government funding have reversed this trend and stifled much important investigative work. If these cuts are not restored, it is absolutely certain that progress will lag. If you are concerned there are only two facts you need to present to your legislator: (1) Health is our most important non-replaceable national asset, and (2) money spent on research is returned a hundred-fold in benefits to society and to the economy.

Following are only a few of the many recent advances in ophthalmology which are already available to help you or someone dear to you.

The laser

Light is one of the most powerful forms of energy in the universe. The light from the sun, 93,000,000 miles away, governs our seasons and, indeed, the life of our planet. The energy from a star, billions of times as far away as our sun, can still be detected by us as a tiny point of light in the heavens.

But powerful as it is, such energy represents only an **infinitesimal fraction** of all the light given off by its source. This is because the energy is not concentrated in a single direction but is diffused. As soon as light leaves its source, the rays are dispersed in **every** direction — dispersed into millions of directions toward **every** point in space — and we see only one or a few of these rays.

Even these few rays have power. They can, with prolonged exposure, cause a sunburn of the skin, or of the retina of the eye. Condensed (focused) by a magnifying lens, they set fire to paper or wood.

Now, imagine if instead of being allowed to spread in **every** direction, a light source could be so controlled that all its energy is sent in a **single** direction. The power of millions of light rays being condensed and concentrated into one ray! This is a laser beam — a beam so powerful that it can cut a hole in a thick steel plate. If the light energy emanating from the sun could be condensed into one beam pointed toward us, it would instantly vaporize the entire earth even from a distance of 93,000,000 miles!

How can a beam of such deadly destructive power be made useful for treating so delicate an organ as the eye? The answer lies in its controllability. Properly designed and in skilled hands, it may be so controlled and focused that the exactly required amount of energy can be delivered to a single, limited microscopic area without harm to adjacent structures.

A high-powered microscope makes surgery with a laser beam even more delicate. Thus it is possible to seal off tiny blood vessels in the retina or the iris where hemorrhages endanger sight. One can seal off, as if by spot-welding, tiny breaks in the retina which threaten to cause its detachment. And without resorting to actual cutting with knife or scissors, one can create an opening in the iris when an artificial pupil is needed. Such procedures can be carried out with a minimum of local anesthesia, or none at all, because the bursts of light, while powerful, are so short (a few milliseconds — thousandths of one second) that they are scarcely perceived by the patient.

Radioactive uptake

One of the by-products of atomic energy research has been our ability to tag certain elements with radioactive substances. In ophthalmology we use a radioactive phosphorus compound which is harmless to the body and which, when injected into the circulation, finds its way into certain kinds of tumor tissue and becomes concentrated there.

If we see or suspect such a tumor within the eyeball, we first inject a minute amount of radioactive phosphorus into the vein of the forearm. We then pass a tiny, sensitive Geiger counter over the surface of the eyeball. An increase in response of the Geiger counter over the questionable area indicates increased phosphorus concentration at that point and helps to reveal the nature of the tumor.

Fooling the virus

Virus diseases are still among the most difficult to cure. Destruction of bacteria by antibiotics is now commonplace. Bacterial diseases that used to kill, or cause months of disability, are now routinely cured by antibiotics, sometimes overnight, with a few injections or pills. Viruses are different. Antibiotics do not touch them. Recovery from most virus diseases still depends on the body's own defenses which are often too slow to build up resistance.

Recently, chemistry has found a way to combat viruses — not by killing them but by fooling them.

The eye, like other parts of the body, is subject to certain virus diseases. One of the most common and most blinding is herpes (pronounced HUR-pees) of the cornea. The herpes virus is related to the one that causes the common cold and also the common cold sore, or fever blister, of the lip or nostril. When it invades the cornea, it causes an ulcer to form on the surface. Worse still, this ulcer does not stand still but grows by branching out in all directions.

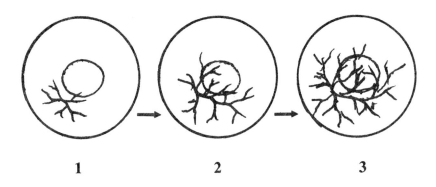

Fig. 9.   Herpes virus spreading over the cornea: 1. early, 2. pupil partly obscured, 3. pupil obscured, vision very blurred.

By the time resistance is marshalled, the branches may have spread far enough to leave permanent scarring and seriously impair the sight. Until chemistry came to the rescue, we used to cure such ulcers (if the patient came early enough) by cauterizing each branch tip with iodine or ether. This was done with the aid of a local anesthetic under a high-powered microscope. Today, we fool the virus with chemistry.

Viruses, like all living organisms, must eat to live. They cause disease by multiplying (reproducing) within our body cells — in this case, in the cells of the cornea. In order to reproduce, their diet must contain certain chemicals. Teamwork among chemists, microbiologists and ophthalmologists succeeded in altering one of these chemicals just enough to stop the reproductive process but not enough to make the virus reject it as a fake! As a result of this chemical "genocide," the virus fails to multiply and dies out.

Today we use these substances, one known by the initials I.D.U. for a long name (iododeoxyuridine), and the other known as Vira-A (Vidarabine), in the form of eye drops and salve which are absorbed by the cornea. If started early enough, before the branching ulcer reaches the central part of the cornea, scarring of the pupil is prevented.

Fluorescein angiography

These big words are baffling until they are taken apart.

Fluorescein is a vegetable dye which, when dissolved, is greenish in color and emits a glow (fluorescence) when exposed to light.

Angiography: "Angio" refers to blood vessels; and "graphy" means "picture of" (as in our word "graphic"). So: "To make a picture of the blood vessels by showing them up with the dye, fluorescein."

Fluorescein angiography is used in special situations

where we need to know more about the flow of blood through the vessels inside the eye.

In the course of a conventional examination with the ophthalmoscope, the circulation of the retina and choroid tells us a great deal about the eye (see Chapter 11). Sometimes this is not enough.

Changes in the vision may be the result of disturbances in the blood flow through these arteries, veins and capillaries — disturbances which cannot be discerned with the ophthalmoscope alone. We can now study the speed and volume of the blood flow by tingeing the blood with minute amounts of fluorescein dye, injected with a fine needle into the vein of the forearm. The eye is not touched, only photographed. Rapid sequence pictures of the back of the eye are taken through the dilated pupil as the dye, flowing with the circulation, quickly shows up the arteries, then the capillaries, and finally the veins.

Where tiny leaks from the capillaries are thus discovered, they can be "spot-welded" with a fine laser beam. This procedure is now commonly applied to arrest hemorrhages in certain diabetic diseases of the retina.

The angiogram requires no hospitalization, no anesthesia and is painless except for a slight prick in the arm. It is not to be confused with the cerebral or the cardiac angiogram. Dye studies of the brain or the heart are totally different procedures which are more serious and involve certain risks. Although many thousands of eye angiograms have been performed, reported reactions to the fluorescein injection have been extremely rare.

A novelty a decade ago, angiography is now routine, although highly specialized and sophisticated. It has enabled us to diagnose and alleviate many conditions whiich formerly resulted in blindness.

Vitreous transplant (vitrectomy)

You have read about removing a cloudy cornea and grafting a clear one in its place (see p. 220), and about removing a cloudy lens (cataract) and even inserting a clear, plastic artificial lens as a substitute (p. 41). It has now become possible, by an operation called vitrectomy, to remove cloudy vitreous and replace it with clear fluid.

The vitreous is the clear, jelly-like fluid which occupies the large space between the lens and the retina (see p. 223 and the drawing inside the cover). Opacity of the vitreous can produce blindness worse than opacity of the cornea or cataract of the lens.

The most common cause of opaque vitreous is hemorrhage from diseased retinal blood vessels, as in diabetic retinopathy (p. 159). It may also result from injury. Vitreous hemorrhages sometimes clear spontaneously. Many fail to clear and new blood vessels then form which make the blindness permanent. Until recently, cloudy vitreous was incurable. Now, in certain cases, vitrectomy restores some vision.

The operation is not suitable for everyone and not all cases are successful. At present we perform it only if the vitreous is very cloudy, if the reduction of vision is severe and if the likelihood of spontaneous clearing is small. In some, the new, clear fluid can again become clouded if the persistent diabetes causes new hemorrhages. When successful, the restored vision is far from perfect but may be enough to enable the patient to get about.

Much research is being done and vitrectomy will surely be improved further. In any case, it brings new hope for those suffering from this once incurable kind of blindness.

Computerized X-Ray

Most people think that X-Rays reveal everything. They

do not. Modern X-Rays will show with great clarity the finest details of **dense** structures such as bone or deposits of calcium. **Softer** tissues, such as muscle, fat, blood vessels, even most tumors, cannot be clearly outlined but appear as blurs.

Some years ago, refinements were made in X-Ray technique — first stereo X-Rays, which, like stereo-photographs, permitted the specialist to get a three-dimensional view. Then, later, tomographs ("tomo" = slice, layer) wherein a series of exposures were made at different **levels**, to view an area in successive "layers." These were improvements, but they still depended on sharp contrast between dense, hard tissue such as bone and lighter, soft tissue.

More recently a bright researcher combined the tomograph (X-Rays in layers) with a computer to give us a very much more sensitive medium, one so sensitive that it can pick out variations and abnormalities even in **soft** tissues.

Successive layers of the skull or of the eye socket are individually X-Rayed to form a composite picture, just as they are in a tomogram, but ever so much finer. The rays activate extremely sensitive elements connected to a computer which transforms each of the thousands of rays into a number. The computer then transforms these numbers into a print-out pattern of light and dark areas which is a map of each "layer." The combination of layers superimposed in perfect sequence, creates a picture of the skull almost as if it were a transparent structure. Because this apparatus is so much more sensitive than X-Ray film to varying **degrees** of density of the living tissue through which it passes, it can distinguish not merely between hard and soft tissues but among varying degrees of softness of tissue. Also, this greater sensitivity means a much lower and shorter dose of radiation than a conventional X-Ray.

And this is but a beginning. Present computerized

X-Rays are at an early stage, comparable to what conventional X-Rays were in 1910. It is only a matter of time before the apparatus is refined to a point where detail will be very much greater than it is now. Already many difficult diagnoses have been made easier. In the brain or in the socket of the eye, for instance, such lesions might formerly have been found only by exploratory surgery or after the injection of air or dye — techniques which involved some discomfort or even risk.

The computerized X-Ray scan, or C.A.T. scan (for Computerized Axial Tomography) as it is known among doctors, requires no anesthesia or special preparation any more than does an ordinary X-Ray. It merely takes a little longer because there are many hundreds of extremely brief exposures instead of a few, but there is no discomfort. Its only drawback is its high cost, over $250, a modest sum when one considers that the apparatus, with computer, costs over a quarter of a million dollars and the annual running expense is almost that much again. Most medical insurance plans probably will cover this soon, if they do not already.

Ultrasound

During World War II, submarine detection (sonar) used the principle of sending high-frequency sound waves into the water to be bounced back off solid objects. The returning sound waves (echoes) were picked up by means of sensitive listening devices. Today the same technique, greatly refined, is used to detect abnormalities within the fluids of the eyeball.

Because the normal pupil is transparent, simply shining a light through it by means of an ophthalmoscope (see Chapter 11) allows the doctor to look in and see abnormalities at the back of the eye. But where the pupil is cloudy, as in cataract or hemorrhage, this is not possible. Just as the patient cannot see **out** of the eye, the doctor cannot see **into** the eye. It is here that ultrasound can detect conditions which would not be visible — tumors, retinal detachments, foreign objects, blood-clots, etc.

This procedure is painless and safe, requires no anesthesia or special preparation, entails no discomfort or risk. In the last few years the technique has been further refined to make it more delicate and more perceptive.

Diagnosis by "Voiceprint"

Fingerprints have long been a standard method of identification. It is commonly accepted that no two people have the same fingerprints. More recently it was discovered that since no two people have identical voices, it is possible to identify a person by matching his "voiceprint."

A voiceprint is the graphic picture of a voice, just as a fingerprint is the picture of the skin ridges in a fingertip. To obtain a voiceprint, a device called a spectrograph translates the sound into a visible wave, then takes it apart and analyzes it into the many waves of which it is composed. Sorting and classifying these many components of sound is a monumental task which only a computer can do quickly and accurately.

If you have read Aleksandr Solzhenitsyn's "The First Circle," you may remember how one of the scientist-prisoners of the Soviet secret police was compelled to work on an invention for identifying people by their telephone voice. This might have been fiction; today it has turned out be fact. The voiceprint can be as unique a signature as a fingerprint.

Recently a Columbia University ophthalmologist, who is talented in physics and electronics and who possesses the imagination of a science fiction writer, decided that if people can be identified by their voiceprints, so can tumors inside the eyeball.

But tumors don't talk! Well, Drs. Jackson Coleman and

Frederic Lizzi make them talk — by bouncing ultrasound waves off them and letting their echo (the reflected waves) become their "voice." They then use a spectrograph and a computer to analyze the echo waves and classify them into their "signature." This signature is fed into the computer's memory bank which compares it with that of other, already "known" tumors. Thus they learn not only the size, location and nature of the growth, but perhaps even its degree of malignancy and its sensitivity to radiation or chemicals. With this information, one may determine what, if anything, will destroy the tumor and cure the patient.

If you think this is pretty wonderful, there's more: this apparatus can see in the dark. Unlike light waves which need a clear pupil, ultrasound waves can penetrate opaque tissue. They can see inside the eye despite a cataractous lens or a vitreous hemorrhage.

And finally there is still more: The same principle which permits ultrasound to penetrate opaque tissue can be used by means of a transducer to focus this powerful but controllable energy on a tumor and possibly destroy it without need for surgery!

Brilliant! But not yet in clinical use as of this writing (1977). With true scientific caution there are hundreds of tests still being done to assure the safety and reliability of the Coleman method. At present, his research team is also storing up a library of signatures of known conditions for purposes of identification, comparison and analysis.

When released for general use this apparatus will be a spectacular step forward toward easier and more accurate diagnosis of hitherto invisible disease within a cloudy eye. Hopefully this apparatus will do even more than locate, see and measure the diseased area; it may, for the first time, be possible to use a beam of sound, instead of a knife, to biopsy (take a sample of) living tissue and perhaps even to destroy a tumor.

15
Choosing an Ophthalmologist

There are two important reasons for choosing your ophthalmologist when you are well — before you really need him. The choice is best made without the stress surrounding an illness or injury. And, when you are ill, his record of your status while healthy will better enable him to compare and evaluate any abnormal condition.

Most people who need an ophthalmologist ask their family doctor or internist to recommend one. Many follow the suggestion of relatives or friends. A call to the local hospital will get you the names of competent ophthalmologists on their staff. Similar information is available by telephoning the medical society whose telephone number is listed under "Medical Society of the County of --------." Some classified telephone books also list doctors by specialty.

Making the choice

When you are at the point of choosing an ophthalmologist, you are really asking yourself two questions: "How competent is he?" and "How concerned is he?"

A doctor's competence depends on his natural intelligence plus his training and experience, all of which enable him to determine what is wrong with you and to cure it, if possible. Concern determines how much effort he will put forth to use that competence in your favor. Lack of competence can be disastrous; fortunately, this is extremely rare, and I'll explain why in a moment. Lack of concern can be anything from bad manners, disagreeable but harmless, to complete heedlessness which could, in extreme instances, be as bad as lack of competence.

Let's discuss competence first; later, we'll talk about concern.

Competence

Medicine is one of the few fields in which standards of training have remained high. In this age of the pampered pupil, any youngster can obtain a high school diploma and almost all can get into college. A great many obtain degrees. But on application to medical school the pampering stops. Most college advisors discourage those not in the top third of their class. Further attrition comes from nation-wide uniform pre-medical admission tests on which many able students score too low for consideration. And this is only the beginning. Out of the many thousands who apply, only the very top ones gain admission. The average class of one hundred entering medical college has been selected from at least a thousand applicants — sometimes five thousand!

The successful ones are given seven to ten years of the most rigorous, the most demanding, the most supervised of all educational courses. The M.D. (doctor of medicine) degree after four years of medical school is merely the half-way mark. It is followed by 4 to 6 more years of post-graduate courses, residency at an eye hospital or in the eye department of a large general hospital and sometimes a fellowship at a similar institution. All aspects of ophthalmology are studied and practiced under supervision: diagnosis, treatment, glasses, diseases and surgery. They must then pass State Board, National Board and Specialty Board examinations. It is impossible to survive all this without ability, devotion and a well-developed habit of hard work.

Consider this from another standpoint — the amount of

sheer time spent learning. After finishing college, from the time he enters medical school until he is ready to practice independently, the average specialist has studied twelve to sixteen hours daily, 300 days a year for eight to ten years — a staggering total of at least 28,000 hours and perhaps as many as 48,000.

I can speak of these men and women at first hand because I have taught many of them. At the eye hospital where I work we have eighteen residents in training, each of whom spends three years with us. In the course of thirty years I have helped train almost two hundred ophthalmologists, usually on an intimate basis: one teacher, one resident. There is no place like an operating room to evaluate ability, judgment, compassion, poise and stamina. Almost all of the two hundred displayed these qualities in abundance and I have every reason to believe that they have retained them now that they have spread out to all parts of the country, most of them as heads of their own departments. I can state categorically that, with very few exceptions, I would allow any of them to operate on me.

The ten thousand ophthalmologists in the country are the product of about fifty institutions, comparable to one at which I have been teaching, all carefully supervised by the American Board of Ophthalmology for top-notch, no-nonsense training.

Following this training they still must be certified by this Board. Having served as an examiner for the Board, I can vouch for the rigorous and comprehensive nature of the tests, both written and practical, that all candidates must pass to be certified as specialists.

Beyond certification there are graduate training courses, clinical conferences and medical meetings which doctors attend all their lives, not only because they want to learn more about the latest developments but also because they are darned interesting.

In addition, medicine is one of the few professions whose members voluntarily subject themselves to self-criticism. For decades past — long before the government mandated peer review — doctors on hospital staffs regularly conducted staff conferences where they review successful and unsuccessful treatments so that they might learn from each other's successes and failures.

Another benefit to the public, of which it is scarcely aware, is the tradition of "no secrecy." There are no secret cures, no secret operations, no secret instruments. Unlike commercial custom, all medical discoveries are freely available to the entire profession. The discoverer is honored for his achievements and is proud to share his knowledge with all doctors everywhere.

Thus, no matter which ophthalmologist you choose, if he is certified and has a hospital staff appointment — which is true for almost all of them — it is virtually certain that he has ability and training and that he has access to all the information available to all the others.

Concern

What about concern? This could be a different matter because you do not have the same safeguards which assure you of competence. Lack of concern cannot be detected among candidates for medical school, nor can it be graded on specialty board examinations. Here you must depend on your own senses, aided, if possible, by the recommendations of your family doctor or those who have had intimate personal contact with the specialist in question.

Yet you do have some real protection — in fact, threefold protection: your own perception of the doctor's attitude, your right to change doctors, and the statistical fact that the overwhelming majority of doctors **are** conscientious.

You need not be extraordinarily perceptive to evaluate your ophthalmologist's concern. Granted your contact is not as intimate as with your family physician, but it is usually possible to distinguish between interest and indifference, between thoroughness and carelessness. But be sure not to confuse speed and efficiency with hurry; some of my colleagues and students complete the same amount of work in half the time that others take. And don't mistake brisk-ness for brusqueness; some will answer your questions concisely and to the point, others like to chat. However, if pertinent and reasonable questions are brushed aside, you are getting less than you have a right to expect.

Your privilege to change doctors is another safeguard. It fits in well with the system of private practice, still available in this country, wherein both the patient and the physician must feel comfortable and satisfied with one another as **individuals**, or else be free to terminate the relationship. Given the reasonable assurance of competence, what patients really want is someone who is interested, someone who cares, who gives them the feeling that "he is responsible for my well-being," and a little deeper down: "I've chosen him because he is concerned." And, at the same time: "He'd better be, because if he isn't, I'll choose some other doctor." This is a healthy state of affairs — good for both patient and doctor.

The third safeguard is in the character of most doctors and in the nature of medical practice generally. With a few glaring exceptions, most doctors **want** to do a proper job — simply because they are proud of their work and their reputation, and willing to labor hard to improve both.

What about the stories of greed, dishonesty, careless-ness, addiction, mental illness? Of course they exist and only a fool would deny it. Doctors, being human, are subject to human failings — perhaps less so for a number of reasons: their work is gratifying and fulfilling, most are too busy for much nonsense, and almost all can earn an adequate living without resorting to dishonesty. In contrast with the thousands who are honest and conscientious, the bad ones are so unusual that they make good newspaper stories. Statistically, your chance of falling into the hands of one of them is small.

In fact, it is favorable rather than adverse publicity which more often confuses the public. Both press and television are eager not only to expose the rare wrongdoer but also prematurely to publicize the spectacular cures which may later turn out a disappointment and lead to recrimination against the entire profession.

Medical directories

Contrary to popular impression, there is nothing difficult or mysterious about looking up any doctor's qualifications in medical directories. The most dependable are the "Directory of Medical Specialists," which is national in scope and lists by specialty all who are certified; and the Medical Directory of your own state which lists all doctors by city. Each doctor's address, telephone number, qualifications, professional associations and hospital appointments are given. One or both volumes are available in most public libraries.

Fees

Again, contrary to popular impression, most doctors' offices are glad to quote their usual or standard fee, even on the telephone, provided there is a "standard." In many instances this is difficult, because no two cases are alike. The secretary cannot know in advance of the visit what procedures and tests will be necessary, in which case only a basic fee may be quoted. Most doctors I know prefer this to having people find out only after the visit. Some offices do not offer this information beforehand unless it is requested, in order to avoid giving the impression that the fee is all that important. When it comes to elective (i.e., non-urgent) surgery, almost all surgeons prefer that their patients know the cost of a given operation in advance and usually urge them to find out hospital charges before they enter the hospital — unless these charges are covered by insurance.

Note: Just published is another book on general health care which is able to devote much more space to "choosing a personal physician." Much of what Dr. Mack Lipkin writes so well about the family doctor in "Straight Talk About Your Health Care" is also applicable to the specialist. I recommend it highly.

16
How the Eye Works:
The Parts of the Eye

Many and varied are the wonders found in nature: the heart, that self-regulating pump which never needs to rest; the brain, a multi-billion-connection switchboard which is more than a super-computer because it not only remembers and calculates, but also thinks and reasons and predicts; the cell, which has a life almost its own and can even reproduce itself; the atom which carries within itself the energy of the universe.

But nowhere in the world is there an organ like the eye, which, in so small a space, combines so many and such varied attributes — usefulness, beauty, clarity, precision, automation, self-focusing, self-positioning, self-adjustment to light, self-maintenance, delicacy and stamina.

You can begin to appreciate the precision of the eye when you consider how much trouble men are taking to duplicate it. Only elaborate instruments many times larger can better discern detail, and these are not as versatile and flexible as the eye. As for self-maintenance and stamina — the eye which is healthy needs no periodic adjustment and will not "wear out" with use, even excessive use, over a long life span. The eye is also a window, a camera and a cable TV as well as the principal pathway to the brain for transmission of knowledge. For the doctor there is an extra bonus: the eye is the only transparent organ in the body. Just as you can see **out** of it, he can see **into** it. The pupil is a peephole through which he can see naked blood vessels and nerves. These tell him much about your general health.

Eyelids and tears

Consider the eyelid, a structure that can be studied just by looking into your mirror. This seemingly simple device is not only the world's oldest windshield wiper but it works perfectly on the **curved** surface of the eyeball. Every motorist has cursed his windshield wiper because it doesn't do a good job on his curved windshield. Yet the eyelid has been doing just that and doing it perfectly for millions of years. Furthermore, with it, as standard equipment, comes a windshield **washer** — the tear gland which manufactures the tear fluid.

Tear fluid in itself is another of nature's marvels. It contains a substance called lysozyme, a powerful germ killer, more potent than carbolic acid yet totally harmless to the eye. (Lysozyme was discovered by Sir Alexander Fleming, the same scientist who years later discovered penicillin.) Without lysozyme the eye would be more susceptible to infection. The tear fluid is produced constantly during your waking hours. The tear gland shuts itself off when not needed, as when the lids are closed in sleep. The amount produced is self-regulated — normally just enough to keep the cornea from drying and to keep the surface of the eyeball moist enough to be slippery. Thus, when the eye moves or when the eyelid blinks, there is no friction between the inner lining (called the conjunctiva) of the eyelid and the front of the eye over which it glides.

Every child knows that tears taste salty. And if you've ever had a tooth pulled or cut your lip you know that blood is salty too. Tears and blood have the same concentration of salt as sea water. Why? Because our ancestors were fish. Millions of years ago, in a much earlier stage of evolution, all animal life existed only in the sea. And that is why our eyes, accustomed to the salt concentration of tears, feel comfortable when we swim in the ocean, but burn and smart when we swim in **fresh** water (even in unchlorinated fresh water). In fact, people who swim a long time in lake water may temporarily experience blurred vision because the cornea, with the same salt content as tears, becomes slightly cloudy from the prolonged absorption of fresh water. This never happens if we swim in the ocean.

In the presence of any irritant, such as a foreign particle, dust, or fumes, the supply of tear fluid is automatically increased. This provides more lysozyme for antisepsis as well as more fluid to dilute and wash away the irritant.

After the tear fluid has done its cleansing, germ-killing and lubrication, it leaves your eye through a tiny drain-pipe, a special tear duct which empties into the nose. That is why your nose "runs" when you cry. You will see the beginning or opening of this duct if you look into a mirror (a magnifying mirror if you are over forty-five) and pull the eyelid a bit away from the eyeball. It is a pinpoint hole on the very edge of the lid near the nasal corner.

The tears do not flow down this duct merely by gravity. They are pumped. Part way down the tear duct, (hidden under the skin near the nose), is a tiny suction pump (the tear sac) which draws the tear fluid out of the eye and down into the nose. This pump is worked by the same muscle that blinks the eye; with each blink it sucks a minute amount of tear fluid from the eye, just enough to keep it from overflowing. The eye "waters" (overflows) when this drain-pipe is obstructed or when there are more tears than the pipe can carry.

Look into the mirror again, this time at the edge of the eyelid. You will see a row of thirty tiny yellowish dots, evenly spaced and just large enough to be visible without magnification. They are the openings of very small glands which lie in the thickness of the eyelid. Each gland manufactures droplets of oil which pass out of the duct to the edge of the lid. This oil coats the lid margin and the lashes just enough to keep the tears, by means of surface tension, within the eye where they belong rather than dribbling down the cheek.

Sometimes the duct of one oil gland becomes plugged, usually by a temporary thickening of the oil itself. The gland keeps on manufacturing the oil but now has no outlet, and so forms a cyst (chalazion). Because the trapped oil has become stagnant, it may become infected, and then is sometimes mistaken for a stye. A stye is only an infection of the root of one of the eyelashes. Both chalazion and stye can be some-what painful and disfiguring but they are harmless and often subside with treatment. They need not be removed unless they get larger or continue to be annoying or ugly. Removal is a minor operation which in adults can be done in the doctor's office under a local anesthetic.

Even the lashes, which help keep insects and raindrops out of the eye, have an intelligence all their own. They grow from roots in the lid margin. The lashes, like all hair shafts, are inert, with no nerves or circulation. They may be cut, as they sometimes are before an eye operation, or they may fall out or be pulled out, but the root always grows another lash. If the shaft of the lash is inert, have you ever wondered how the root knows when to stop making the lash longer?

By far the most marvelous and most important of all mechanisms connected with the eyelid is the blink reflex. This lightning-quick reaction is triggered by anything which might harm the eye, whether it be an object which is seen approaching, or an irritation which is felt. In milliseconds (thousandths of a second) the warning is flashed by a nerve to the brain and back, and the lid is closed, usually in time to protect the eye or to wipe off a particle by its windshield-wiper-like action. Without the protection of this reflex, the eye could easily be injured and become cloudy. In fact, if the lid loses its ability to blink, as in certain kinds of nerve disease or injury (facial paralysis, Bell's palsy), it may be necessary to wear a glass or plastic shield over the eye to protect it and to prevent it from drying.

Lastly, one of the most important attributes of our eyelids is the ability to close them and shut out the visible world. Think what this means to our sleep, our rest, our privacy and our sanity. Consider what life would be if, like our ears, our eyes were incessantly open.

How nice if we also had **ear** lids. Perhaps, in another million years of noisy environment, man will evolve ear-lids, too, and be able to shut out rock music, traffic and jet noise, the telephone — and the alarm clock. A bit risky, perhaps, because one of the senses must stand guard.

Now this is but a sample of the simplest and most apparent part of the visual apparatus. If your curiosity has been aroused, you may come with me inside the eye on a guided tour. Such a tour must be brief, and often so oversimplified as to verge on inaccuracy. (A standard complete book on the same subject fills twelve large volumes for a total of over 20,000 pages, comprehensible only to one who has been through medical college.) A guided tour is always better understood when one has a map. For convenience, you will find one inside the front cover.

The cornea and sclera

The cornea is to the eye what the crystal is to a watch — and much more because it is a living thing. The tough, but delicate and sensitive outer coat of the eye consists of two parts, the cornea and the sclera. The cornea is clear as crystal and is situated in front of the pupil and iris. The sclera is opaque and protects the rest of the eye — it is seen in the mirror as the "white of the eye." The cornea is so clear that unless you look closely you are not even aware of its presence. Most people think the pupil and the colored iris are the **front** of the eye. It is only after their attention has been alerted that they see them as **behind** the cornea, as the face and hands of a watch lie **behind** the crystal.

The cornea is perfectly clear because its fibres are in precise alignment. Any interference with this orderly alignment makes the cornea cloudy and blurs the vision. This can happen as a result of disease, injury or scarring. If the clouding is in the very center of the cornea, (the part in front of the black pupil), the impairment of vision may be severe and permanent. Because it is so vulnerable to injury and permanent clouding, the cornea is protected by its great sensitivity — it is one of the most sensitive structures in the body. Its surface is richly supplied with delicate and invisible nerves which respond to the slightest touch or threat of a touch, by calling into play the other protective mechanisms, the blink reflexes and the lid. The blink instantly wipes off anything which lands on the cornea; the closing of the lid protects it from harm.

Anything happening to the cornea causes acute pain which warns us to get help. Loss of this sensitivity or loss of the blink reflex or of the lid action makes the cornea vulnerable to injury. (The subjects of injury and foreign objects are dealt with in Chapter 8 on injuries and the prevention of blindness. Contact lenses, which fit on the cornea, are discussed in Chapter 13.)

Corneal Transplants

Should the clouding of the center of the cornea be severe enough, particularly if it involves both eyes or the only good eye, it is now quite possible to remove the cloudy center and graft a clear cornea into its place. This is one of the most delicate and dramatic operations in all surgery and is usually successful in restoring the vision. It is painless, can be done at any age under either local or general anesthesia. The only difficulty is the need for a donor, one who donates an eye so that its healthy, clear cornea can be grafted in place of the patient's cloudy one.

Fortunately, American research and organization have found a solution to the donor problem, but much depends on the cooperation of the public. Research workers have discovered that the donated eye need no longer necessarily come from a live donor but may be obtained from someone just deceased.

Anyone can bequeath an eye. The only requisite is prompt, signed consent by the next of kin as soon as death occurs. This is certain to be a shocking concept if it is first broached to the survivors at the moment of bereavement. But it is totally sensible and natural if discussed candidly among family members while all are in good health and the prospect of death, though inevitable, is remote. Sentiment yields to common sense when a prospective donor realizes that his corneas become useless when he dies, but if donated, they literally continue to live on, giving the precious gift of sight to some adult or child who would otherwise have remained blind.

Anyone who agrees with this — and who could not? — can arrange to bequeath his corneas by simply advising his family and by registering with the local Eye Bank or with the Eye Bank for Sight Restoration, 210 East 64th Street, New York City, 10021, on the tenth floor of the Manhattan Eye, Ear and Throat Hospital. There is nothing final about such an arrangement because you can cancel it at any time. In addition, to be valid it still requires the signed consent of the next of kin promptly after the donor's death. And there is no disfigurement whatever in the appearance of the deceased after such a donation has been made.

There is never any expense to either donor or recipient,

both of whom remain anonymous. All costs are met by the **Eye Bank** which is a non-profit organization supported by private contributions, large and small. Local eye institution personnel handle the medical aspects of the donation and the local Red Cross provides ground transportation. Where necessary, the airlines give first priority to flying donated material quickly to any part of the country where the surgical team is waiting to operate on the patient whose sight is to be restored by a new, clear cornea.

The conjunctiva

Starting at the edge of the cornea and covering the white of the eye is a thin, transparent membrane called the conjunctiva. Extending backward on the eyeball behind the upper and lower eyelids, it doubles forward to line the lids, so that the two surfaces of the conjunctiva (that covering the white and that covering the inside of the lids) glide over one another when the lids blink or when the eye moves. To prevent friction, the conjunctiva contains tiny glands which manufacture mucus. The mucus combines with the ever-present tear fluid to make a lubricant — a lubricant so slippery that you are not aware of any friction when the eye or the lids move.

When you view your eye in the mirror, you do not see the conjunctiva because it is so thin and transparent that you look right through it and see only the white sclera behind it — just as you must look twice at the iris and pupil to realize that the clear cornea is in front. It is only when you search more carefully that you note the tiny blood vessels which are barely visible in the conjunctiva. When the eye is inflamed for any reason, these vessels become much more prominent and make the eye look red. (See Chapter 9 on ''The Inflamed Eye.'')

The fluids of the eye

Once past the cornea, we are inside the eyeball and all the structures we now encounter are immersed in fluids. The eyeball is filled with two kinds of fluid — the front portion in the narrow space between the cornea and the lens contains the aqueous, or watery, fluid; the back portion, the relatively large space between the lens and retina, contains the vitreous, a fluid which has a gelatin-like consistency. These fluids do more than fill out the eye to keep it from collapsing, they carry nourishment and other vital substances such as antibodies (germ fighters) from the blood to the intra-ocular structures and are part of a fascinating mechanism for maintaining the correct pressure within the eye. Disruption of this mechanism causes a disease known as Glaucoma, to which all of Chapter 2 is devoted.

The iris

The iris is the organ which gives the eye its color. Like the skin, the color of the eye depends on the amount of pigment it contains. People with fairer skin have less iris pigment and their eyes are usually blue or light grey. Darker skins are usually associated with heavily pigmented brown or black eyes. Absence of pigment in eye or skin is rare — such people or animals are known as albinos. An albino eye looks pinkish because of the reddish tinge of light reflected from the rich blood supply lining the inside of the eye.

The most important function of the iris is performed by two tiny muscles which regulate the size of the pupil. One muscle surrounds it like a purse-string. When it contracts, it makes the pupil **smaller**. The other radiates outward from the pupil in all directions like the petals of a daisy. Its contraction makes the pupil **larger**.

The pupil

The pupil is not really a structure. Actually it is merely a hole in the iris. The normal pupil is black because the lining of the eye is pigmented and black, like the inside of a camera. The pupil, by contracting and dilating, regulates the amount of light permitted to enter the eye, and does so automatically with marvelous speed and precision. When light enters the eye, a nerve impulse notifies the brain. It tells the brain not only that there is light, but it also measures the amount of light, like a light-meter, and conveys this, too, to the brain. Via another nerve, the brain instantly flashes back instructions to the tiny muscles within the iris, telling them how much to contract or expand the pupil.

Perform this experiment — look at your own pupil in a mirror using dim light. Then turn a flashlight on your own eye. You will see your pupil contract. When you turn off the flashlight, the pupil dilates again. Then repeat the experiment with a small light and again with a very bright light and note the difference in the amount of pupillary contraction.

Besides reacting to light, the pupil is affected by other stimuli, such as emotions, by certain drugs or poisons, or by focusing of the eye for near vision. With age, the pupils tend to become somewhat smaller; in childhood they are larger, sometimes enough to alarm a mother so that she telephones the doctor, only to be reassured that this is often normal in children. If instructed to flash a bright light into the eye, she will observe that the child's pupil contracts normally.

Abnormalities of the pupil occur in certain medical disorders as well as in some brain diseases or injuries. Thus, observation of the pupil is important not only to the eye specialist, but also to the general doctor, the internist, the neurologist and the emergency room physician. In sleep, the pupil is usually smaller; in death, it is dilated. Patients using drops for glaucoma usually have small pupils, as do morphine and heroin addicts when they have taken the drug.

Sometimes the eye specialist uses drops to enlarge the pupil in order to examine the interior of the eye more easily or to measure the amount of far-sightedness or astigmatism more accurately. This is a harmless procedure (if the eye pressure is normal), but it may cause temporary inconvenience from inability to focus or from the entrance of too much light. (Sunglasses worn on leaving the office will help.) The additional wait in the office for the drops to take effect can be irksome, but it is done to save you another visit. So be prepared to spend more time if necessary.

After dilating the pupil, the doctor may use other drops to contract it again. This may cause a different kind of discomfort: a slight cramp-like sensation in or above the eye, or a feeling of dimness (if the pupils become too small and let in too little light.). Either or both reactions are harmless and last only a few hours.

What holds the lens in place
(the ciliary body and the zonule)

Just back of the iris, behind its outer edge and therefore not visible from in front, is a small, dark, ring-like structure called the ciliary body. (For this and other structures described here, see Fig. 10, page 227.) A circle of tiny spider-web-like fibers, the zonule, or the zonular fibers, stretches from the ciliary body to the lens and holds it in place.

In addition to the task of focusing the lens (we will learn how, a few pages further on), the ciliary body also manufactures the clear aqueous fluid which fills the anterior chamber, the space between the cornea and the iris. This watery fluid gives the eye its shape by keeping it full under just the right amount of pressure. It also has the function of bathing the lens, the back of the cornea and the front of the vitreous — a very important function because none of these three structures has its own nourishing blood vessels. (The presence of blood vessels would spoil their perfect clearness.) It is the aqueous which transmits to them the substances necessary for their survival — salts, sugars, antibodies (germ killing substances). These chemicals, in minute, precisely regulated amounts, are cleverly withdrawn from the blood vessels of the ciliary body by microscopic pumps and mixed with the aqueous. In certain diabetics, a rise in the sugar content of the blood becomes a rise in sugar content of the aqueous which changes the focusing power of that fluid enough to make the eye more far-sighted. Alerted by such a finding during a routine eye examination, I have, on many occasions, been able to discover early diabetes which had not been suspected by the patient because there were as yet no other symptoms.

The aqueous fluid does not just sit stagnant in the anterior chamber. This life-giving nutrient has a circulation all its own — in fact, two circulations: one an inflow-outflow, the other a slow churning within the chamber. You may find this hard to believe, but in the tiny space between the cornea and the iris the fluid circulates on the same principle as does water in the ocean — the cold moving downward and the warm, upward! If you look at the side-view diagram of the anterior chamber, you will see that the front, next to the cornea is cooler than the back which is next to the iris, one of the warmest places in the body (because, second only to the thyroid gland, it has the richest blood supply in the body).

The arrows in the diagram depict the direction of circulation, the aqueous cooled by contact with the cornea flows downward while that warmed by the iris, rises.

The other circulation — inflow and outflow — is even more important. The aqueous, newly formed in the ciliary

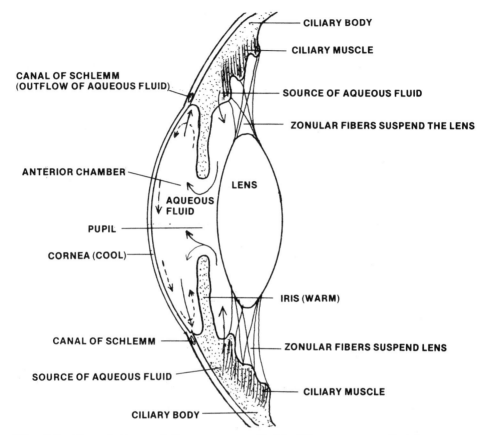

FRONT OF EYEBALL (SIDE VIEW)
(FOR ORIENTATION, SEE INSIDE OF FRONT COVER)

Fig. 10. Circulation of the aqueous fluid. The aqueous fluid flows in two currents: Inflow-Outflow (solid arrows) and Convection (dotted arrows). The **inflow** starts at the ciliary body. Here the aqueous is derived from the blood vessels which supply the aqueous with nutrients and antibodies destined for the lens and the cornea. The aqueous flows forward through the pupil into the anterior chamber (solid arrows). There the **convection** currents (dotted arrows) churn it so that the nutrients are distributed. The fluid then leaves the eyeball via the tiny **outflow canal** (the canal of Schlemm) carrying waste products to be reabsorbed into the blood vessels.

body, enters the anterior chamber through the pupil, is caught up and mixed by the churning action just described, and finally leaves the chamber through a tiny drainage canal called the Canal of Schlemm.

This marvelous mechanism does more than distribute nourishment and antibodies in the eye and carry waste material out. It also adjusts the volume of outflow by a series of incredibly sensitive microscopic controls, which balance it exactly against the amount of fluid being produced by the ciliary body.

Thus, the pressure of the fluid within the eye is kept at exactly the correct level. Any disturbance of this adjustment can lead to increased pressure, known as glaucoma, a condition so serious that we devote a full chapter to it (Chapter 2).

The lens
(Accommodation)

The lens is one of the most intriguing structures in the body because it can change its shape to focus the eye. You have just read how the lens is suspended directly behind the pupil held in place by the zonular fibers (see Fig. 10, p. 227). These delicate fibers stretch from the edges of the lens to the tiny but powerful muscles within the ciliary body. At the command of a special nerve coming from the brain, the contraction of these muscles tightens or loosens the zonular fibers. This pull, transmitted to the lens — which is flexible! — changes its shape just enough to focus the eye for distance or for near or anywhere in between. The act of focusing is called "accommodation."

With age, usually beginning around forty, the lens becomes progressively less flexible and therefore more difficult to focus. Consequently older persons need increasingly stronger reading glasses to do the focusing for an eye which is still normal but no longer able to focus itself. This is called "presbyopia" (presby = old; opia = eye). There are more details about lenses, glasses and how the eye works in Chapter 17.

In older people the most important disease of the lens is cataract. This is so widespread that I have devoted all of Chapter 3 to it.

The choroid

Lying between the sclera and the retina is a very important structure called the choroid (pronounced KOH-royd). It consists of a maze of blood vessels, large and small, plus millions of microscopic capillaries. The blood in these capillaries brings nourishment to the sensitive part of the retina which contains the rods and cones. Without this blood supply there would be no sight.

The retina

The retina is to the eye what the film is to the camera, and much, much more. Like the film, it lines the back of the eye and receives the image focused on it. Here the similarity ends, because it also acts as the transmitter of that image to the brain, which translates it into the realm of the owner's awareness. Unlike a film which is used only once for a single image and discarded, the retina keeps on renewing itself, is used millions of times by constantly changing images, and is never discarded but lasts a lifetime.

This marvel of sensitivity and organization is made up of many millions of receiving cells, sending cells, connecting and supporting cells. Receiving cells are of two kinds: you've probably heard of **rods and cones**, so named because that is their shape when viewed under a microscope. They not only look different, but they see differently.

The **cones** provide the sharply detailed sight — the sight you use when you read fine print, sew a fine seam or read a distant street sign, the kind of vision you need to score 20/20 on the vision chart. Such sharpness is possible because most of the millions of cones are packed tightly in a tiny area at the center of the retina (the **macula** — see the diagram inside the front cover), and because each one of these millions of cones has its own private connection (nerve fiber) via the optic nerve to the brain.

So important is the macular area that, although it is only a millimeter in diameter, less than one percent of the entire retina, the nerve fibers from it make up more than 60% of the optic nerve.

Two kinds of vision

But this is not to say that the other 99% of the retina is unimportant. It is extremely important in a different and very special way. It does all the seeing of everything but the center. This is called **peripheral** vision, in contrast to vision at the center (the macula), which is called **central** vision.

Peripheral vision is performed by the **rod** cells which are not concentrated in the center like the cones, but are scattered all over the rest of the retina. Unlike the cones, they do not have individual nerve connections to the brain, but many rods share single nerves. For this reason peripheral vision is not as sharp as central vision. Instead, it has two other capabilities — it is better able to detect movement of objects which are not directly ahead, and it is better able to see in dim light. Both of these functions were more important a few million years ago when no animal, human or otherwise, could have survived if he had not been able to spot an approaching enemy. They are still important in such activities as driving if you consider other cars as "enemies" from whom you need protection.

To understand peripheral vision, perform this simple

experiment: Look straight ahead of you with your line of sight fixed on one object in the room. Now, without moving your eyes, note all the other objects in the room which are visible although you do not look directly at them. This is the precious peripheral vision which you have been taking for granted all your life. Then, for contrast, take a sheet of letter-size paper and roll it up into a hollow tube about an inch in diameter. Hold one end up to your eye like a tele-scope, pressing this end of the tube gently against the surrounding eye socket: close the other eye. You are now looking with only your central vision and with practically none of your peripheral vision. Stand ten feet away from your television screen or from a newspaper; you can see the screen or read the headline very well but can see nothing on any side of them! This is referred to as "tunnel vision" or "telescopic vision." Now try walking about the room and you will quickly realize the importance of peripheral vision and how helpless you would be without it.

Can you imagine driving a car with no peripheral vision? Or even with defective peripheral vision? There are some people who do, especially those with late glaucoma, many of whom are not aware they have the disease! (See the case history of Mr. Williams at the beginning of Chapter 2.) There are states which require only good central vision for a driver's license; other states test peripheral vision as well.

So now you have seen that you really possess **two** kinds of vision. **Central** vision is necessary for detail, **peripheral** for getting about, for orientation within your environment, and for protection.

Speaking of peripheral vision, have you noticed that "hunted" creatures like rabbits, deer, most birds and others which are preyed upon by flesh eating animals, have their eyes on the **sides** of their heads? This gives them almost 360 degrees or a full circle of peripheral vision — practically 'eyes in the backs of their heads,' and enables them to detect an enemy approaching, even from behind.

Most hunting animals do not have this facility and do not need it as much. They, like us, have their two eyes in front, which gives them "**binocular**" (**two**-eye) vision and **depth perception** — the ability to judge distance so that they can accurately gauge their jump when they stalk their prey — a fascinating subject which we will touch on presently.

So, with our two eyes to the front, what we gain in having binocular vision we lose in peripheral vision. Instead of seeing almost a full circle (360°) like the squirrel, we are able to detect motion in only a bit more than half a circle (about 190°).

Just as there are diseases like glaucoma which impair the peripheral vision, so there are those of the macula which impair the central vision. The latter occur occasionally in older persons, in certain disturbances of circulation affecting the tiny blood vessels of the eye, and sometimes as the result of tobacco smoking or of staring at the sun during an eclipse. This condition is discussed more fully in Chapter 11 on your eyes and your health, and also on p. 131.

A Few More Interesting Facts About The Retina

Color blindness

The retina is also the seat of color vision. This is mostly the function of the cones, and color vision is therefore better near the center than at the periphery.

Most color blindness is an inability to distinguish between green and red. This is usually a recessive hereditary characteristic which is sex-linked, occurring in about 8% of all males, but is transmitted by the female. Thus, the children of a color-blind father are not themselves color-blind, but his daughters are likely to transmit this trait to their sons. Thus the defect skips a generation and affects alternate generations of males.

One would think that in our world of color, this would be a great handicap. In actual practice, color-blind people get along quite well. Although there is no cure, those who are not profoundly affected learn to accommodate and compensate, though they find it difficult to perform tasks in which color discrimination is critical.

People who are color-blind are rarely aware of it until it is pointed out to them. A minor part of the eye examination of young boys consists of color testing with charts specially designed to detect color defect.

Night blindness

You have learned that the rods in the periphery of the retina see better than the cones in the dim light. Defects of the rod cells or disease in the periphery of the retina causes an inability to see well in dim light — known as night blindness.

Conversely, the cones see better in good light and more poorly in dim light. Try this experiment: On a dark night, look at the sky and pick out a star which is so tiny that you can just barely see it. Now, if you fix your gaze intently (with your macula) on such a star, it disappears. If you then shift your gaze a hairsbreadth away from it (meaning you are now using a part of the retina just outside your macula), the star becomes visible. This shows that the cone cells in the macula do not function in darkness.

In fact, if cones are kept in darkness for long periods of time, they permanently lose their ability to see! In olden days, total and permanent loss of central (cone) vision was common among prisoners kept in dark dungeons for long periods of time and among miners who worked seven days a week and never saw daylight because they were always below ground from before sunrise to after dark. There are cases on record of refugees from the Nazis before and during World War II who lost central vision as a result of long periods of hiding in dark cellars.

Loss of retinal function can also result from deprivation of **Vitamin A**. When a retinal cell reacts to light, one of its chemicals, a substance called rhodopsin, is bleached and momentarily made useless. Its restoration to the unbleached state — ready to work again — depends on the presence of Vitamin A. Total absence of this vitamin in the diet is extremely rare in this part of the world, but, when it happens, vision can be impaired. However, it takes very small amounts of Vitamin A to supply the retina's needs — supplied by any ordinary sensible diet or perhaps by the equivalent of half a carrot a day.

This does not mean that there is any advantage in consuming large quantities of carrots. More than the small amount needed will not make ordinary vision any better, nor will it improve vision which is defective for other reasons. Occasionally I have come across patients who have erroneously reasoned thus, some of whom have gone to such extremes that their skins turned yellow from excessive carotene pigment.

For detachment of the retina, see Chapter 4.

Eye movements

The eyes of almost all mammals move within their sockets, but in humans the range of motion is greater. Much has been written about survival factors in evolution, such as the opposable thumb and coordination of eye and hand. Less attention has been paid to the fact that the greater mobility of the eyes has contributed substantially to man's ability to manipulate, to learn and to survive. Think how much more difficult it would be to work with your hands if your eyes did not move within their sockets and you had to turn your head for every change in direction. Think how hard it would be to read under such circumstances.

The eyes do more than just move in every possible direction. They do so in perfect coordination **with one another**. This coordination not only allows us to keep moving objects in view, it achieves a function, binocular vision, which becomes more than the sum of its parts.

Depth perception

One eye alone is capable of doing almost everything a pair of eyes can do — except judge distance. True judgment of distance, also referred to as "depth perception," "three-dimension vision," "stereoscopic vision" or "stereopsis," requires not only two eyes ("binocular vision"), but both working together as a team.

Try this experiment:

Place any person with two good eyes so that he is opposite you and so that you can see his eyes clearly. Ask him to look through the window at a distant object, then switch his gaze to the window sash. You will observe that in the second position, his eyes move toward one another (converge) ever so slightly. Now switch his gaze to your finger held nearer to his face. His eyes will converge still more — minutely but noticeably. Now let him look back to the distance and you will see his eyes straighten.

More important, not only can you see the tiny convergence and divergence but **he** can **feel** the adjustment himself. It is this **sensation** which, unconsciously and automatically, enables him to judge whether one object is nearer or further than another.

The eye muscles

Each eye has its own six muscles. Four are called

"rectus" muscles (rectus is Latin for "straight"), which draw the eye upward (superior rectus), downward (inferior rectus), toward the nose (medial rectus), and outward (lateral rectus). The remaining two are called "oblique" muscles because they tilt the eye obliquely. Varying degrees of action among these six muscles turn an eye toward any point in space. Each muscle is controlled by its own nerve which originates in a switching center in the mid-brain. That center is activated by several relays of other nerves coming from higher command and consciousness centers in the brain. Complex sets of connections link these nerves with other centers which control movements of the head, the body, the limbs and the balancing mechanism in the inner ear. Still other relays act to make the two eyes work as a pair. Any disruption of these delicate switching arrangements interferes with the coordination of the two eyes and causes double vision.

Double vision

People sometimes complain of **double** vision when they really mean **blurred** vision, or, conversely they may describe it as blurred when it is in reality double. Either symptom is potentially serious in its own right and demands attention. But you will help the ophthalmologist make an accurate diagnosis more promptly if you keep the two symptoms straight.

Blurring is a haziness or lack of clarity of outline, an indistinctness as of a picture which is out of focus; it may be experienced with one eye alone or with both together.

Double vision means literally: two separate images seen when both eyes are used at the same time but not well coordinated. The two images may be separated horizontally (side by side), vertically (one above the other) or obliquely, depending on how the muscles fail to balance. The double vision may be constant or intermittent, and the images may be very close together in which case they can be very annoying, or so far apart as to be scarcely noticeable. Another test of whether it is really double vision is that it can be eliminated by closing either eye.

Many normal people can make themselves see two images by forcing their eyes **not** to coordinate. Try this experiment: Hold your finger or a small light about twelve or eighteen inches before your face, look at it, then look past it as if you were focusing at something across the room. The finger or light will appear double. Now re-focus your eyes on the object and it becomes single again. In fact, if you are observant you may catch sight of the two images in the act of merging back into one.

Occasionally, older people experience transient double vision especially while looking at distant objects. The further the object, the more the two images separate. The exact cause of this is not known; it is thought to be a minor disturbance in circulation. Some patients may be relieved by wearing a special lens containing a prism which helps to fuse the two images into one.

But double vision can sometimes be a danger signal. It may come from disease of the brain, of the circulation, or from certain poisons. The specific list of possible causes would take many pages and would be pointless and confusing here. Suffice it to say that anyone with double vision ought to have an examination by an eye specialist. Only an eye specialist, sometimes in consultation with an internist or a neurologist, can determine its nature, its cause, its seriousness and its treatment. Double vision which develops suddenly, especially if persistent and accompanied by general malaise, headache or nausea is urgently in need of prompt examination.

17
How the Eye Works: Focusing (Refraction)

In order to see properly, the normal human eye must perform two basic tasks: 1. focus the image on the retina, 2. transmit the retinal image to the brain.

We have already discussed how light stimulates the retina and how the image is transmitted via the optic nerve to the brain. But merely seeing a blurred image is not enough. The vision of humans and most animals must also be sharp (in focus). In addition, the picture projected upon the retina must be made so small that an entire panorama can be compressed into less than a square inch of retina — something on the order of a space-satellite photograph which reduces a whole continent to the size of a picture post-card. The eye does this easily, quickly and automatically, employing the structures in front of the retina: the cornea, the aqueous fluid, the iris with its pupil, the lens with its ciliary body, and the vitreous (see the diagram inside the cover). The technical term for this process is "refraction."

Refraction

The word "refraction" is used to describe any process related to changing the direction (focusing) of light rays. It comes from the same word as "fracture" meaning to break, i.e., to alter the straightness, thus, to bend (to bend a ray of light). We speak of the refractive power of an eye or of a lens, such as a spectacle lens. "Errors of refraction" are the result of slight defects in the focusing power of the eye, such as far-sightedness, near-sightedness, astigmatism. They may be corrected by lenses in spectacles worn before the eye or by contact lenses worn on the eye (in contact with it), properly ground to neutralize the error. The science of measuring the eye for glasses is also called "refraction."

Refraction is easy to understand if you learn how a light beam can be bent. A beam of light is a column of light rays, all parallel to one another, travelling in a straight line. In outer space, where it meets practically no resistance, it moves at 186,000 miles per second. When it strikes the earth's atmosphere, it is slowed a bit. On entering a substance like glass or the eye, it is retarded even more, because glass or the eye are denser than air.

When the beam strikes such a transparent (denser) surface not head-on, but **obliquely**, its nearer rays reach that surface sooner than other rays, causing the beam to change its direction just as a car, speeding on a concrete road, swerves if one wheel strikes a sandy stretch which slows it up.

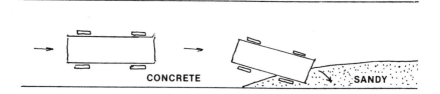

Fig. 11. A car swerves when one wheel strikes a different surface. This illustrates the principle of refraction.

A classic example is the column of soldiers marching on a firm pavement coming upon a slower terrain, like sand. Those reaching the sand first would be slowed up, while the others still on firm ground would keep up their normal gait, causing the marching column to be deflected.

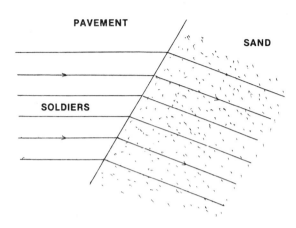

Fig. 12. Columns of soldiers deflected as they reach a change in footing.

Now if, instead of lines of soldiers deflected by the change in footing from concrete to sand, you substitute rays of light bent by the change from air to a slower medium like glass — you have "refraction."

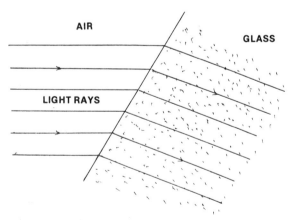

Fig. 13. Light rays bent as they pass through from air to the slower medium of glass.

Carry this a bit further and let the light rays emerge from glass back into air. If the glass is wedge-shaped, like a prism, the rays will be bent still more.

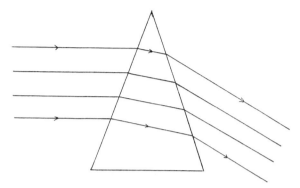

Fig. 14. A prism bends the light as it enters and emerges from the glass.

Now take **two** prisms, placed base to base, and each one will bend rays toward its base so that they converge (focus).

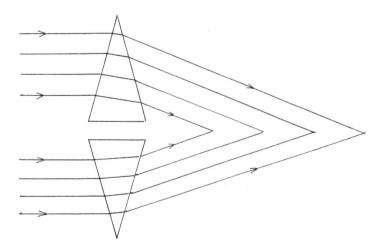

Fig. 15. Two prisms, base to base, can focus light rays.

A convex lens is almost like a pair of such prisms, but with curved surfaces instead of straight ones.

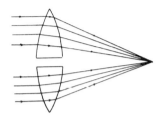

Fig. 16. A convex lens, which acts like two prisms.

Each of the two surfaces acts to bring the rays to a focus. The first surface (front of the lens) converges the rays a little, the second surface (back of the lens) converges them more. The more sharply curved the two surfaces of the lens, the more will the rays be converged and the closer to the lens will be the point where all the rays meet (the focus). (See also Fig. 24, p. 246.)

The eye has **three** focusing surfaces, each of which converges the rays a little more:

       1. the front curved surface of the cornea.
       2. the front curved surface of the lens.
       3. the back curved surface of the lens.

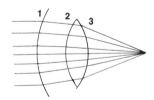

Fig. 17. The three focusing surfaces of the eye.

Now you understand how the cornea (1) and the lens (2,3) cause the rays to converge to a focus. If we fill in the rest of the eye (dotted line), you will find that this focus falls on the retina (4).

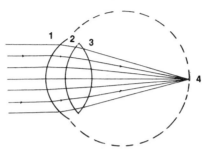

Fig. 18. Light rays focused by the lens and cornea to a point on the retina.

Before we go to far-sighted and near-sighted eyes, I will digress for a moment to speak briefly of lenses. There are two basic kinds of lenses, convex and concave. A convex lens converges the light rays in the same way as the cornea and lens of the eye converge them.

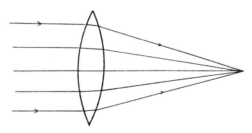

Fig. 19. A convex lens converges light rays.

A concave lens diverges the light rays which pass through it. A concave lens is thinner in the center than at the edge. The name is best remembered if you think of it as being hollowed out like a "cave" (con**cave**).

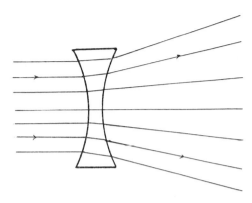

Fig. 20. A concave lens diverges light rays.

The convex lens is also technically known as a "plus" (+) lens and is used in far-sightedness and presbyopia (see below). The concave lens is also called a "minus" (-) lens and is used in near-sightedness.

Errors of refraction
Far-sightedness, near-sightedness, presbyopia, astigmatism

Most human eyes are constructed very much alike — with two minor exceptions: slight differences in total length of the eyeball and slight variation in the curvature of the cornea.

We have just seen how, in a normal eye, parallel light rays coming from a distance are bent toward one another so that they all meet (focus) on the retina (see Fig. 18). This is correctly focused vision, and is called Emmetropia.

Some eyes are shorter. In these the rays would focus behind the retina because the retina is too far forward. These are called far-sighted (Hyperopia). (See Fig. 22, opposite.)

Some eyes are longer and the focus would be in front of the retinal because the retina is too far back. They are near-sighted (Myopia). (See Fig. 23, opposite.)

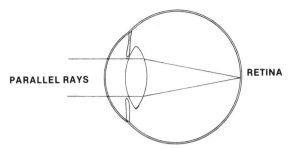

Fig. 21. Normal (Emmetropic) eye. The eyeball is just the right length. Parallel rays focus on the retina.

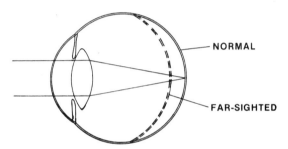

Fig. 22. Far-sighted (Hyperopic) eye. The eyeball (dotted lines) is too short. Light rays focus behind the retina.

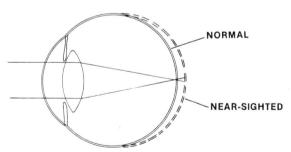

Fig. 23. Near-sighted (Myopic) eye. Eyeball (dotted lines) is too long. Light rays focus in front of the retina.

Correction of far-sightedness

In the far-sighted eye we have seen that distant (parallel) rays would come to a focus too far behind the retina. To bring the focus forward on to the retina (see the dotted lines), the lens within the eye makes itself more curved (more convex, stronger — see dotted curve).

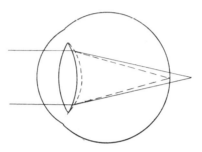

Fig. 24.   Correction of far-sightedness by the lens of the eye itself.

Or, this may be accomplished instead by placing a convex glass in front of the eye.

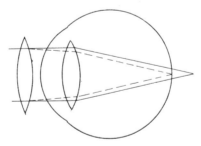

Fig. 25.   Correction of far-sightedness by a convex lens placed in front of the eye.

Here, the added glass lens does the additional focusing, relieving the lens within the eye of the need to do so.

Correction of near-sightedness

In near-sightedness (myopia) we have the opposite problem. The myopic eye is **longer** than normal and the focus falls **short** of the retina. Far objects (parallel rays) are out of focus.

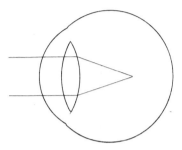

Fig. 26. A near-sighted eye without correction.

A **concave** lens, worn in front of the eye **spreads** the rays instead of condensing them, and thus moves the focus back so that it falls upon the retina.

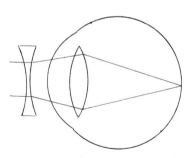

Fig. 27. Correction of a near-sighted eye by a concave lens.

How the eye changes focus (accommodation)

Even the simplest camera must have two kinds of adjustment: variable focus, and variable light. So does the eye:

Light (brightness) is regulated by automatic change in the size of the pupil as described on page 224.

Focus is changed by the lens which has the almost magic ability to adjust its focusing power by changing its shape at the command of the brain. This act is called "accommodation" — the eye accommodates itself to the new focal distance. When we try to look at an object close by, it is out of focus. A signal is sent down the nerve to the tiny muscles in the ciliary body (see Fig. 10 page 227). Contraction of these muscles changes the amount of pull on the zonular fibers which hold the lens suspended in position. This pull increases the curvature of the lens because (up to middle age) it is soft and flexible.

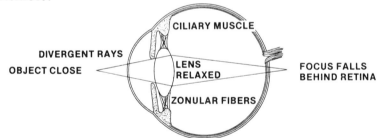

Fig. 28. Before accomodation: Divergent rays from a close object are focused by relaxed lens at a point behind retina.

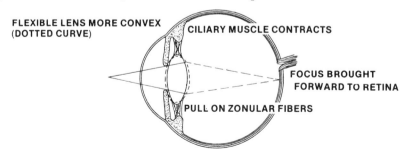

Fig. 29. Accomodation: Flexible lens makes itself more convex, converges rays more. Focus comes forward to retina.

You will get an idea of the extreme delicacy of this adjustment when you realize that in shifting the focus from print held two feet away to print held one foot away, the change in the thickness of the lens is measured in thousandths of an inch. Even more wonderful is the control (again via other nerves from the brain) which coordinates the focus of the **two** eyes **simultaneously** so that their images are equally clear!

Presbyopia

In childhood the lens is soft and flexible, making accommodation very easy and prompt. With age this flexibility diminishes and by the mid-forties the normal eye may have difficulty focusing print at reading distance. It is at this age that normal people begin to need reading glasses to do the focusing which the eyes can no longer do. This is called "presbyopia" (presby = old; opia = sight).

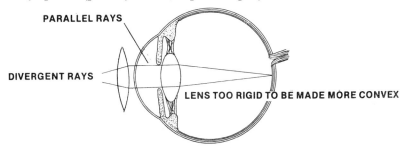

Fig. 30. Accomodation impossible because of age: Lens is too inflexible to make itself more convex to focus rays from a close object. A spectacle lens converges the rays to parallel before they reach the lens, which focuses them at the retina.

This loss in flexibility becomes gradually more pronounced requiring a change in reading glasses each year until about sixty-five or seventy when it levels off. Thereafter, little or no change is required.

Many people are alarmed when their near vision becomes progressively poorer and they need stronger glasses each year. They think they are beginning to go blind. They are relieved to learn that this is a normal phenomenon and that with proper glasses, they may, if their eyes are otherwise healthy, continue to read fine print as long as they live.

Astigmatism

Astigmatism is a bit more difficult to grasp. You must try to visualize the eye as the three-dimensional globe it is, rather than the two-dimensional (flat) circle which is the only way it can be drawn on paper. The cornea is not a segment of a circle   but a segment of a sphere (like a watch crystal).

If it were a perfect sphere the curvature would be the same in all directions and there would be no astigmatism.

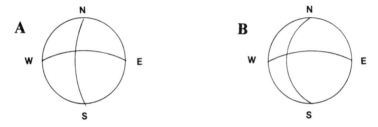

Fig. 31.   **A**: N-S meridian **same** curvature as E-W.
          B: N-S meridian **more** curved than E-W.

But let the North-South meridian of the cornea (N-S), for example, be more sharply curved than the East-West (E-W), the rays from the one will not be focused on the same **spot** as the rays from the other. A-stigmat-ism therefore refers to the condition in which there is **no spot** at which the rays come to a focus (a = no; stigma = spot). This failure to focus can be corrected by putting before the eye a special lens (astigmatic lens) which compensates for the disparity in the curvatures of the cornea. Another way of correcting the astigmatism is by wearing a contact lens. By substituting the uniform surface of the contact lens for the irregular surface of the cornea, all the rays are made to converge on a single point of the retina.

Keratoconus (conical cornea)

There is a special, more extreme kind of irregularity of the cornea in which the shape, instead of being a segment of a sphere, becomes slightly cone-shaped.

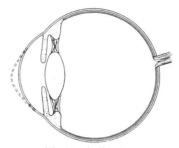

Fig. 32.   Conical cornea (dotted line).

A powerful astigmatic spectacle lens may correct a slight degree of keratoconus. If the cornea becomes more conical, such a lens may not be sufficient and a contact lens may be necessary. In more extreme conditions, it requires a corneal graft to achieve acceptable vision. Fortunately, the great majority of corneal graft operations are successful. (For more on corneal graft, see p. 220.)

A word about lenses

We have already seen how a **convex** lens **converges** light rays to a **closer** focus and how a **concave** lens **diverges** rays to move the focus **further** away, and that lenses are ground in different strengths. Convex lenses are expressed as "plus" (+) lenses and concave as "minus" (-), and the strength is expressed in Diopters. A diopter refers to the focusing power of a lens. In convex lenses, **one** diopter is the strength required to converge parallel light rays to a point **one** meter away, and is written + 1.00 D.   The 2 diopter (+ 2.00 D.) lens is twice as strong and focuses twice as close, i.e., **half** a meter.   The + 4.00 D. lens is four times as strong and so focuses at one quarter of a meter. The + 10.00 lens focuses ten times as close as the + 1.00 lens, i.e., 1/10 meter.

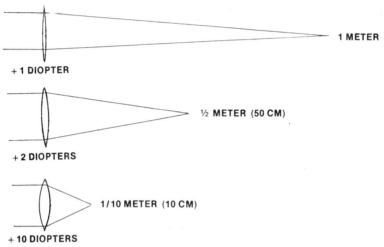

Fig. 33. Focal lengths of three lenses.

If a person is far-sighted enough to require a + 1.00 D. lens for distance and an **additional** + 2.50 glass for near, his glasses would be as follows:

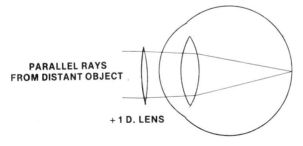

Fig. 34. A far-sighted eye requiring a + 1 D. lens to make **parallel** rays from **distant** objects focus on the retina.

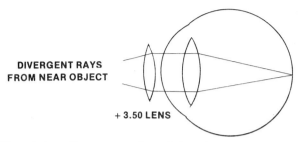

DIVERGENT RAYS
FROM NEAR OBJECT

+ 3.50 LENS

Fig. 35. The same far-sighted eye requiring an additional + 2.50 D. lens to focus **divergent** rays from **near** objects. The total correction is (+ 1 D.) for far + (+ 2.50 D.) for near = + 3.50 D.

Bifocals and trifocals

Those whose work requires frequent and repeated change of glasses from distance to near and back again may prefer to wear **bifocals**, which are nothing more than distance correction at the top and near correction at the bottom, fused into one lens.

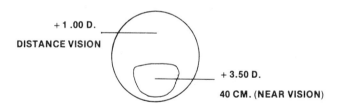

+ 1 .00 D.

DISTANCE VISION

+ 3.50 D.

40 CM. (NEAR VISION)

Fig. 36. A bifocal lens with a correction of + 1.00 D for distant vision and + 3.50 D. for near vision (40 cm.).

There are some who require more than bifocals, as for example a violinist who plays in a symphony orchestra. He may want to wear **trifocals:**

+ 1.00 to see the conductor

+ 2.50 to read the music on his stand 66 cm. away

+ 4.00 to read newsprint at 33 cm.

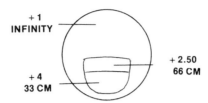

Fig. 37. A trifocal lens has segments for three distances.

There is nothing mysterious about bifocals or trifocals. They are merely means of combining two or three lenses into one. This obviates the necessity of constantly changing glasses.

There is a popular superstition that if you have bifocals you are obliged to wear them constantly. This is simply not true. Like any other glasses, wear them only when you need them, that is, only when you need to see better — distance **and** near — or if you experience discomfort when you remove them.

You may be puzzled by the difference in the shape of bifocal reading segments.

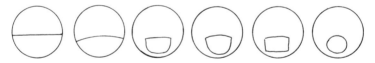

Fig. 38. Variations in shapes of bifocal reading segments.

I usually leave that choice to your optician because he has the expertise to evaluate which type is best for your particular purpose. He makes the decision depending on the prescription, the best curve of the new lens, the curve of your old lens, the difference between the correction of the two eyes, the type of work you do and the type of bifocal you have already been wearing, if any. This is important because there is often temporary discomfort after switching to an unaccustomed type. It may mean **un**-learning an old habit and learning a new one, of redirecting the gaze when shifting from distance to near and back again.

Frames

Another important consideration is the height of the junction line between the distance and reading segments. The optician adjusts this by fitting your frame carefully. All new bifocal or trifocal wearers mind this dividing line at first but almost all rapidly acclimate to it. The rule is that the segment must sit exactly right for the task at hand. If the top of the segment is too high, it may interfere with your looking ahead in the distance; if too low, you may be forced to tilt your head back or else hold your book too close to your chest in order to read.

The frame must fit well and snugly. Obviously, if the frame keeps slipping down or forward, the reading segment will never be in the same place twice, especially for those who wear their glasses constantly and walk about with them.

Base curves

You recall I mentioned the curve of the lens. Each glass has a front curvature and a back curvature. These are called the "base curves." The difference between front and back curves is what gives the lens its "strength" or focusing power. Lenses may be ground on different base curves and still have the same strength. For example: comparing the three lenses drawn schematically in cross section:

Lens A is ground on a front curve of "plus 6" and a back curve of "minus 4." Their sum is "plus 2" ($+6-4=+2$). Lens B is on a front curve of "plus 3" and a back curve of "minus 1." The sum is the same "plus 2" ($+3-1=+2$). The lens C, the sum is $(+1)+(+1)=+2$.

If the prescription calls for a "plus 2," all three of the above will be correct. But if a sensitive person has, for a year or two, worn a +2 as shown in lens A, and switches to the same +2 as shown in B or C (the correct lens but an unaccustomed base curve), he may be uncomfortable for a few days or a few weeks until he has become accustomed to the new curve.

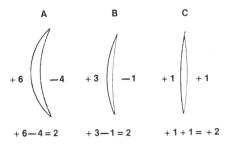

Fig. 39. Lenses of the same strength (+2 D.) may have different base curves.

Index

About the Author

As a practicing eye specialist for over a third of a century, the author is familiar with the problems of patients, their anxieties, and how to answer in simple terms the questions they most frequently ask.

Dr. Esterman is Consulting Ophthalmic Surgeon at the Manhattan Eye, Ear and Throat Hospital in New York City. He has served as Attending Ophthalmic Surgeon at that hospital and at the New York Hospital—Cornell Medical Center. He is Director Emeritus of Ophthalmology at the hospitals on Long Island where he practices: Peninsula Hospital Center, the South Shore Division of St. John's Episcopal Hospital and the South Shore Division of the Long Island Jewish Hospital.

Dr. Esterman holds degrees from Columbia and, with honors, from the Cornell University Medical College. Most of his residency training was under Dr. Arnold Knapp at the Herman Knapp Memorial Eye Hospital, now merged with the Eye Institute in New York City.

He is a Fellow of numerous medical societies, national and international, past president of the New York Society for Clinical Ophthalmology and, in 1967, received an award of the American Academy of Ophthalmology for his work on peripheral vision. He was co-founder in 1938 of the world's first glaucoma clinic, an institution which has since become standard in every eye hospital.